Regina Augustine

Keep Moving!

Keep Moving!

It's Aerobic Dance
SECOND EDITION

Esther Kan
SOLANO COLLEGE

Minda Goodman Kraines
MISSION COLLEGE

Mayfield Publishing Company

Library of Congress Cataloging-in-Publication Data

Kan, Esther.
    Keep Moving! : it's aerobic dance / Esther Kan, Minda Goodman
Kraines. — 2nd ed.
        p.   cm.
    Includes bibliographical references and index.
    ISBN 0-87484-990-X
    1. Aerobic dancing.   I. Kraines, Minda Goodman.   II. Title.
    RA781.15.K36   1991
    613.7'15—dc20   91–22628
                                                              CIP

Manufactured in the United States of America

10 9 8 7 6 5 4 3

Mayfield Publishing Company
1240 Villa Street
Mountain View, California 94041

Sponsoring editor, James Bull; managing
editor, Linda Toy; production editor,
Carol Zafiropoulos; manuscript editor,
Andrea McCarrick. This text was set in
9 1/2/11 Garamond by Carlisle Communi-
cations and printed on 50# Finch
Opaque by Malloy Lithographing.

Contents

Foreword

Keep Moving! It's Aerobic Dance is an excellent book for anyone interested in fitness. I've been teaching Aerobic Dance since 1976. It has been my pleasure and reward to watch it grow into a multi-million-dollar-a-year industry . . . You can't stop a good program!

Naturally, in any field that is growing at such a tremendous rate, it is difficult to keep participants well informed. That is what this book aims to do—provide good, up-to-date information.

Esther Kan and Minda Goodman Kraines have produced a well-written, practical, and educational book—truly one of the best I've read on the subject. They completely break down all the elements of aerobic dance, from why an aerobic workout is important to what the various components of an aerobic dance class are. This includes movement tips, how to add variety to your workout, precaution boxes so you can avoid injury, and even a glossary to help you learn and remember important aerobic dance terms. Nutrition, body composition, components of fitness, and much more are addressed in *Keep Moving! It's Aerobic Dance*.

Joanie Greggains
"Morning Stretch"

Foreword

Your personal lifestyle choices, experts say, greatly affect your health. For a long and healthy life, you need to maintain an ideal body weight, avoid smoking and substance abuse, watch your intake of saturated fats and salt, and include substantial amounts of fruits, vegetables, and fiber in your diet. Above all, you need exercise. With its intrinsic benefits and its ability to moderate many risk factors, exercise is the key to your personal health program.

At first inspection, these new prescriptions for a healthy life may seem terribly limiting and disagreeable. But no perception could be further from the truth. Health requires autonomy, personal independence, voluntary selection of options, and assumption of the power to change your own future. Good health allows you to freely experience joy, beauty, and triumph.

In this book, written with both joyous expression and scientific accuracy, Esther Kan and Minda Goodman Kraines provide the feeling as well as the substance of an important form of exercise that can help you achieve good health. Aerobic dance can help you control many specific risks to good health and at the same time provide enjoyment in its purest sense. *Keep Moving!* provides a solid, scientific background necessary for the beginning student of aerobic dance to understand what happens to the body during the early months of aerobic training. Description of the warm-ups and dances will help the beginner become familiar with unfamiliar exercises and routines that are the basis of a successful dance program.

I liked this book very much in the first edition. Now, it is even stronger and better. The chapter on introduction of variety is useful—we want lifetime aerobics. Sections on low-impact aerobics and avoidance of nagging injuries further will help keep exercise a long-term part of your life. Many other chapters and improvements have been added.

I hope that many will read and use this book and embark successfully on new experiences.

James F. Fries, M.D.
author of *Take Care of Yourself, Taking Care of
Your Child, Aging Well,* and *Comprehensive
Guide to Arthritis*
Associate Professor, Stanford University School
of Medicine

Preface

We have been extremely gratified by the success of the first edition of *Keep Moving!* Since its publication in 1987, more than 50,000 college students have found it an invaluable resource for getting the most out of their aerobic dance classes.

Our goals remain the same in this second edition: To provide lucid, accurate coverage of the basic scientific and physiological principles that underlie aerobic dance; to describe the most popular aerobic dances clearly and with an abundance of illustrations; and to offer brief discussions of such vital topics as injuries, nutrition, stress, posture, and flexibility so that class time can be spent dancing.

The second edition of *Keep Moving!* offers the following features:

- Completely revised and updated coverage of the important scientific and physiological principles that underlie aerobic dance;
- Clear, well-illustrated descriptions of dozens of popular, contemporary aerobic dance movements. *Keep Moving!* includes more than 300 how-to illustrations;
- A new chapter on nonimpact and low-impact aerobics (Chapter 9);
- More than thirty precautions boxes that help students avoid injury;
- Movement tips, which have been added to help students master particularly challenging dance moves;

- Two chapters on the important cool-down phase of the aerobic workout (Chapters 10 and 12);
- A new chapter on how to add variety to your aerobic workout (Chapter 16);
- Three new appendixes, covering video cassette workouts (Appendix E), music resources (Appendix C), and answers to frequently asked questions (Appendix A);
- A separate chapter on what to expect in an aerobic dance class (Chapter 5);
- A new glossary to help students learn and remember important aerobic dance terms.

Minda Goodman Kraines wishes to thank her husband, Guy Kraines, and her daughters, Denaya and Marissa. Without their love and support she could not have completed her work on this book. Esther Kan would like to thank Mariam Combs for her assistance and encouragement.

We would like to express our appreciation to those who served as models for the illustrations in this book and on the cover: Christopher Anasco, Lisá Marie Austin, Prescillo Baltar, Robin Bertz, Guillermo Garcia, Kelly Garcia, Michael Kan, Julia Kimsey, Stuart McGee, Patrice Rackstraw, Antonio Silva, and Karen Stenger. Special thanks also to Karin Bivens and Phil Sienna.

We would like to thank the following reviewers for their valuable suggestions: Maridy Bronstein, University of Alabama; Elizabeth Brown, University of Maryland; Lisa Rene Chaisson, Lamar University; Christine Cobb, Youngstown State University; Gwen English, Wright State University; Gail G. Evans, San Jose State University; Lorna L. Francis, San Diego State University; Barbara Jahn, University of California at Davis; Janine McAlpin, Lorain County Community College; Beverly McCraw, Duke University; Janice Gudde Plastino, University of California at Irvine; Karin Volkwein, University of Tennessee, Knoxville; Donna Wilson, Southern Illinois University at Carbondale; Penny Wright, Tarleton State University.

Keep Moving!

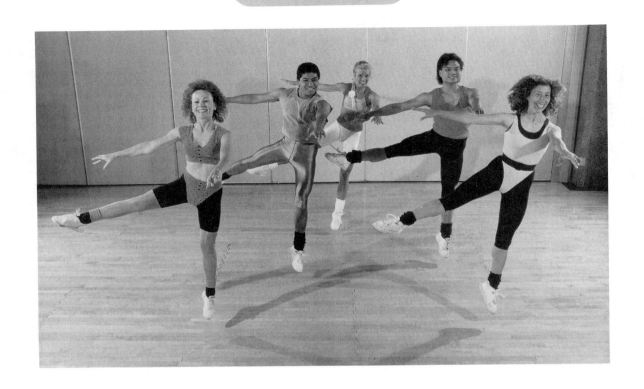

What Is Fitness?

Chapter

The term *fitness* is broadly used and often vaguely defined. Many people perceive health and fitness as one and the same, yet there is a definite distinction between the two concepts. Health reflects a person's state of being; it is typically viewed as the presence or absence of disease. Fitness, on the other hand, is the ability to do physical activity or to perform physical work (29).

Health and physical education experts generally agree about the expanded (but incomplete) definition of fitness as an ability to carry out daily tasks with vigor and alertness, without undue fatigue, while still maintaining ample energy to enjoy leisure-time pursuits and to meet unforeseen emergencies.

Although not scientifically proven, it is generally agreed that fitness makes a major contribution to a healthier, longer, and more productive life.

Characteristics of a healthy lifestyle include regular exercise, a nutritious diet, and plenty of rest and relaxation. But what actually is the definition of fitness? What aspects are important for a healthy body? To define fitness we must understand the terms *strength, flexibility,* and *endurance*. It is the combination of these three components that leads to the achievement of fitness.

STRENGTH

Strength is the ability of a muscle or a group of muscles to exert force. Maximal strength is when a group of muscles exerts a force against a resistance in one all-out effort (32), such as one maximum lift in a weight-lifting exercise.

The body needs muscular strength for several reasons. First, strong muscles increase joint stability, which in turn makes the body joints less susceptible to injury (32). Second, improved muscle tone also helps prevent common postural problems. For example, stronger abdominal muscles can help alleviate postural problems associated with the lower back. Often, lower back problems occur because the strength in the spinal muscles is greater than that in the abdominal muscles; this muscular imbalance causes the postural deviation **lordosis** (swayback). Weakened muscles of the upper back can cause the postural deviations termed **kyphosis** (rounding of the upper back) and/or round shoulders. By building strength in the weakened muscles, these postural deviations may be modified or alleviated. Finally, the body needs muscular strength because it contributes to agility, helps control the weight of the body in motion, and helps the body maneuver quickly (32).

In developing muscular strength, the muscles must be contracted against a heavy resistance with a minimum of exercise repetitions. It is important that minimum repetitions and maximum resistance be used in order to improve muscular strength. Many repetitions with light weights will not increase muscular strength. As the muscles become stronger, the resistance applied must be increased (32) if muscular strength is to continue to increase.

FLEXIBILITY

Although **flexibility** is generally associated with the elasticity of muscles, the total concept of flexibility is denoted by the range of motion of a certain joint and its corresponding muscle groups. Flexibility is influenced by the structure of the joint's bones and ligaments, the amount of bulk that surrounds the joint, and the elasticity of the muscles whose tendons cross the joint (32).

The range of motion of the body's various joints is called *joint mobility.* Joint mobility is measured by the amount of movement that exists where two joint surfaces articulate with each other. The greater the range of motion at the joint, the more the muscles can flex and extend. This range of motion or joint mobility is specific to each joint in the body. For example, your hip joint may be extremely flexible, whereas your shoulder joint may be inflexible (42).

There are several reasons why good joint mobility and muscular elasticity should be maintained. The movement range of muscles and joints not used frequently and regularly throughout their full range of motion becomes limited. Many movement experts claim that a lack of flexibility is a cause of improper movement performance in simple motor activities such as walking and running (32). Good joint mobility and muscular elasticity can also increase resistance to muscular injury and soreness; it is the person with inflexible muscles and joints who may experience muscular soreness or who may be more easily injured during activity because of the limited range of motion (32). However, too much flexibility in certain joints—such as the weight-bearing joints of the hips, knees, or ankles—may make a person more susceptible to injury or hamper performance. Loose ligaments may allow a joint to twist abnormally, tearing the cartilage and other soft tissue. In general, it is advisable to achieve and maintain a "normal" amount of flexibility throughout the body. Normal range varies with each individual.

For flexibility to be increased, the muscles must be stretched beyond their normal range of motion for at least 10 to 30 seconds (15). As flexibility increases, the range of the stretch must also be increased for continued improvement in flexibility. An in-depth discussion of proper stretching techniques are discussed in Chapter 12.

ENDURANCE

Endurance is the ability of a muscle or group of muscles to perform work (repeated muscular contractions) for a long time. With endurance, a muscle is able to resist fatigue when a movement is repeated over and over or when a muscle is held in a static contraction (the muscle generates a motionless force for an extended time) (22).

There are two types of endurance: muscular and cardiorespiratory. **Muscular endurance** is the ability of local skeletal muscles to work strenuously for progressively longer periods of time without fatigue, such as during the execution of 50 sit-ups. Note that muscle endurance is highly specific; it will be attained only by the specific muscles exercised (32).

Using light weights and doing many repetitions of an exercise will increase muscular endurance. This task will tone the muscle but, unlike strength building, will not create large muscle bulk. Increasing muscular endurance is often termed *body sculpting,* or *body toning.*

The other type of endurance is **cardiorespiratory endurance.** This is the aspect of fitness that involves the heart and the lungs—the most important muscles of your body. Cardiorespiratory (also called cardiovascular) endurance is the ability of the cardiovascular system (heart and blood vessels) and the respiratory system (lungs and air passages) to function efficiently during sustained, vigorous activities, such as running, swimming, and cycling. To function efficiently, the cardiorespiratory system must be able to increase both the amount of oxygen-rich blood it delivers to the working muscles and its ability to carry away carbon dioxide and other waste products.

To enhance cardiorespiratory endurance through exercise, the activity must fulfill certain criteria. It must be of sufficient intensity, duration, and frequency; involve large muscle groups; and be continuous, rhythmic, and repetitive. These criteria are termed *intensity, duration, frequency,* and *mode.* Without their proper application, cardiorespiratory endurance will not improve. Activities that adhere to these guidelines are termed **aerobic** activities. Walking, jogging, running, swimming, biking, cross-country skiing, stair climbing, trampolining, and, of course, aerobic dance are all aerobic activities.

Aerobic Exercise versus Anaerobic Exercise

To fully understand aerobic exercise, we must define the energy systems that occur in the body and how the energy from these systems is utilized for movement. In order for the muscles in our body to contract, which is necessary for movement, a substance termed **ATP** (adenosine triphosphate) must be present in the muscle cell. The initial burst of energy for muscular contraction requires no nutrients or oxygen. This energy system is called the **phosphagen system,** named after the compound **creatine phosphate,** which

exists in the muscle cell. Creatine phosphate breaks down the ATP to release energy for immediate muscular contraction. Since there is a limited amount of ATP that is always present in the cell, this energy system can contract the muscles for only 10 seconds or less. At the end of that time, either nutrients or oxygen must be delivered in order to resynthesize the ATP for continued muscular contraction. A vertical jump or maximum weight lift are examples of activities utilizing the phosphagen energy system.

After the initial burst of energy, the nutrient **glycogen** (the storage form of glucose) that is present in our muscle cell is used to continue the resynthesis of ATP. Like creatine phosphate, there is a limited amount of glycogen stored in our muscles. The supply of glycogen present in a muscle cell can continue muscle contraction for up to 2 minutes. The energy system that uses only the stored glycogen in our muscle cells to resynthesize the ATP is termed *anaerobic glycolysis.* Anaerobic means "without oxygen," and glycolysis refers to the breakdown of glycogen (a form of carbohydrate). This energy system, like the phosphagen system, is only used for intense bursts of energy. Windsprints or ten repetitions of a bench press are examples of activities utilizing this energy system.

Unlike the phosphagen system, which has no end product, anaerobic glycolysis produces **lactic acid.** As lactic acid builds up in the cell, the muscle will fatigue and muscular contraction will become increasingly more difficult. You have probably heard the term "going for the burn." This burn occurs when oxygen cannot be delivered to the cell to adequately meet the needs of the working muscle. At this point, the anaerobic energy system has been depleted and the aerobic energy system starts to function. Oxygen must now be supplied to the muscle cells in order for muscular contraction to continue.

Along with oxygen, nutrients are also needed to continue the resynthesis of ATP. The initial phases of aerobic exercise will utilize the nutrient glycogen—the same nutrient that was used in anaerobic glycolysis. When exercise continues for 20 minutes or more, fat will also be utilized to resynthesize ATP to continue muscular contraction.

General Characteristics of the Energy Systems

Characteristic	System		
	PHOSPHAGEN	**ANAEROBIC**	**AEROBIC**
FUEL	Creatine phosphate	Carbohydrate (glycogen)	Carbohydrate and fat
AMOUNT OF ATP PRODUCED	Very little	Limited	Unlimited
END PRODUCTS	None	Lactic acid	Carbon dioxide, water
OXYGEN REQUIRED	No	No	Yes
DURATION	0–10 seconds	10 seconds–2 minutes	2 minutes and beyond
TYPE OF ACTIVITY	Sprint or high power, short duration	High intensity, up to 2 minutes	Moderate intensity, long duration

As long as oxygen and nutrients reach the cell, movement can be continued indefinitely because, unlike anaerobic glycolysis, the only end products of aerobic exercise are water and carbon dioxide, both of which are passed through the body. This makes aerobic exercise the most efficient means for improving the fitness of the cardiorespiratory system. It is this ability of the heart and lungs to deliver the oxygen and nutrients to the muscles to resynthesize ATP that determines an individual's success in aerobic activities. (See the chart above for a comparison of the energy systems.)

TRAINING EFFECT

The term *training effect* refers to the physiological changes that occur in the body due to regular and proper participation in a fitness program. To build a healthy body, participation in fitness activities is essential. However, unless the exercise is performed safely and effectively, the results may be minimal. To achieve a training effect and experience the benefits of exercise (whether strength, flexibility, or endurance), the individual must apply the concepts of (1) threshold of training, (2) the overload principle, (3) progression, and (4) the specificity principle.

Threshold of Training

In developing physical fitness, there is a "correct" amount of exercise that will produce effective conditioning results. The **threshold of training** is the minimum amount of exercise necessary to produce improvements in physical fitness. The *fitness target zone* is within the threshold of training and the point where the benefits of exercise become counterproductive (see Chapter 3). To get optimal benefits from regular exercise, a person should exercise within the fitness target zone. Each component of fitness—strength, flexibility, and endurance—has its own threshold of training and fitness target zone. In addition, to gain fitness, a person must "overload" above the threshold of training for the exercise performed (15).

Overload Principle

For a person to experience a training effect, selected systems of the body must be subjected to loads greater than those to which they are accustomed. This is known as the **overload principle:** A body adapts to the higher performance levels and gradually increases its capacity to do more work. The principle can be summed up in this simple "rule": Do a little more today than you did yesterday, and do a little more tomorrow than you did today.

The overload principle affects the development of strength, flexibility, and endurance. For muscular strength to increase, muscles must work against a greater-than-normal load. For flexibility to increase, muscles must be stretched beyond their current length. For endurance to improve, muscles must be exposed to increasingly longer sustained work. For cardiorespiratory endurance to improve, there must be an increased demand on the heart and lungs to sustain aerobic activity.

Basically, the overload principle may be applied to a fitness program in five ways:

1. Increase the number of repetitions or distance of the exercise.
2. Increase the duration or time of the exercise.
3. Increase the speed of the exercise.
4. Increase the intensity or resistance of the exercise.
5. Decrease the rest intervals between exercise.

For the cardiorespiratory system to attain a training effect, three variables of overload must be applied to the training program: intensity, duration, and frequency.

Intensity

Intensity refers to how stressful the exercise is. In the cardiorespiratory system, the intensity of the exercise should correspond to approximately 60 to 85 percent of a person's maximum heart rate (3). Exercise performed at a level below 60 percent of the maximum heart rate offers few, if any, conditioning benefits. Similarly, activity at levels above 85 percent provides little added benefits and, in fact, may be dangerous for some people.

Duration

Duration is the length of each exercise session. For cardiorespiratory fitness to be developed, exercise should be 15 to 60 minutes of continuous activity, the time depending on the intensity of the activity. Lower intensity activities must be performed for a longer time and are recommended for the nonathletic adult (3).

Frequency

Frequency is the number of exercise periods each week; 3 to 5 sessions a week are necessary for a training effect to be achieved (3). Even exercise of adequate intensity and duration may not effectively improve physical fitness if it is not performed regularly (3).

A minimum of 8 to 12 weeks is necessary for a training effect to result. Thus, even if the intensity, duration, and frequency are sufficient, most likely there will be no cardiorespiratory changes unless there has been participation in a continuous program for a minimum of 8 weeks.

Progression

Progression goes hand in hand with overload. When overload is applied to the workout, it must be done progressively, or a little bit at a time. When overloading the duration of an aerobic workout, the principle of progression would add 3 to 5 minutes on to the workout once the initial workout had reached a comfortable state. Applying progression to intensity and frequency works the same way; once the exercise has achieved a comfortable state, slightly increase the intensity or add another day to the workout regime. Never go from 2 days to 5 days all at once or 20 minutes to 40 minutes in one workout. Although the progression principle may appear to be a rule of logic and common sense, it is sometimes overlooked. Failure to adhere to a sound principle of progression may result in unnecessary soreness and/or injury.

Specificity Principle

The **specificity principle** (specific adaptations to imposed demands—SAID—principle) is a unifying concept that applies to all areas of fitness. It means that the human body adapts specifically to the demands placed on it. For example, strength training induces specific strength adaptations, but strength training does *not* develop cardiorespiratory fitness. Only training involving aerobic exercises produces specific endurance training adaptations (38).

The specificity principle also applies to each body part. If the legs are exercised, fitness is built in the legs. If the arms are exercised, fitness is built in the arms. For example, male gymnasts involved only in apparatus events may have good upper body development but poor leg development (15). Finally, the specificity principle applies to certain activities—specificity of training. Specific exercise elicits specific adaptations, creating specific training effects (32). Training is most effective when it closely resembles the activity for which a person is training (15), using the specific muscles involved in the desired performance (38). For example, for an individual to improve the performance of the shot put, the person must perform both an exercise that overloads the arm muscles and a training motion that closely resembles the motion of the shot put (15). Whatever you are trying to achieve, you must train your body specifically for that outcome.

FITNESS FOR LIFE

To maintain a healthy lifestyle, every individual must be fit. You should be physically fit enough so that you can meet the needs of your occupation and daily activities and still be able to enjoy leisure-time activities at the end of a day. By being physically fit, you can gain maximum benefits from your body. As John F. Kennedy said, "Physical fitness is not only one of the most important keys to a healthy body, it is also the basis of dynamic and creative activity."

Why not start now to make your fitness and health a lifetime concern? Physical movement is stimulating and refreshing. There are many types of and variations to exercise programs; you should select one that meets your personal interests and needs. The most important decision, however, is to choose to exercise regularly, *for life*. This book should motivate you to enjoy the fun of exercise through aerobic dance. Wait no longer. Read on to see how you can start walking, stretching, hopping, running, and jumping your way to fitness.

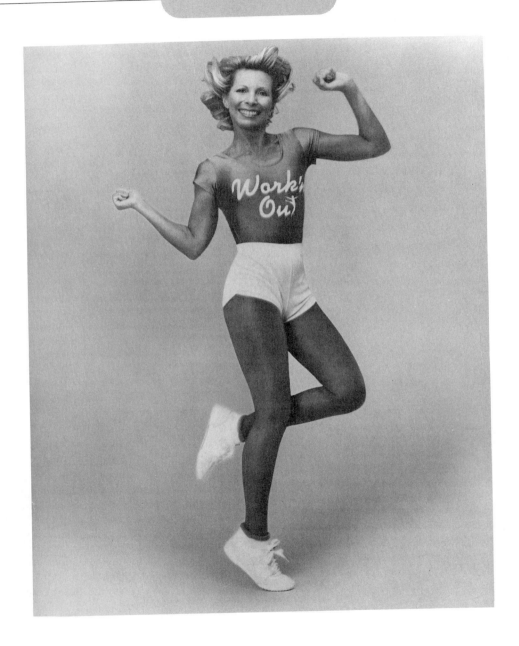

Jacki Sorensen, founder and creator of Aerobic Dance.

Why the Aerobic Workout Is So Important

Chapter 2

Cardiorespiratory fitness is the most important element of physical fitness because it enables the cardiorespiratory system to carry on its functions efficiently under conditions of heavy work and physical stress. An efficient cardiorespiratory system is able to deliver large amounts of oxygen-rich blood to the working muscles over extended periods of time. The format of an aerobic dance class is designed to increase the efficiency of the heart and lungs by incorporating nonstop rhythmic exercises that demand large amounts of oxygen. Thus, regular participation in an aerobic dance class is one of the best ways to improve your cardiorespiratory system.

BODILY CHANGES DURING A WORKOUT

To fully appreciate the value of an aerobic conditioning program, you should understand what happens to your body during the aerobic dance class and the importance and benefits of the workout. The obvious bodily changes that occur during a workout are sweating, heavier-than-normal breathing, and fatigued muscles. The internal effects from aerobic exercise are not visibly apparent; the heart, lungs, blood vessels, and the body's metabolism all undergo changes.

Heart

During an aerobic workout, both the rate at which the heart beats (heart rate) and the amount of blood the heart pumps per beat (**stroke volume**) increase so that the total amount of blood the heart pumps in 1 minute (**cardiac output**) increases. Blood pressure is also affected by aerobic exercise. **Systolic blood pressure,** a measure of the rhythmic contraction of the heart as blood *leaves* the heart via the ventricles, rises with increased cardiac output. **Diastolic blood pressure** is a measure of the resting pressure in the arteries when the heart is not contracting. This blood pressure usually remains the same or slightly decreases during the course of aerobic exercise (32, 36, 38).

Lungs

During aerobic exercise, the body demands more oxygen, so the lungs must deliver more oxygen to the working muscles through the blood. In turn, excess carbon dioxide must be removed from the muscles through the blood. For this accelerated exchange of oxygen and carbon dioxide between the lungs and the blood to occur, both the rate and the depth of breathing must increase (36).

Blood Vessels

During aerobic exercise, the blood vessels shift the blood flow from the visceral (abdominal) organs to the working muscles and to the skin. The muscles of the body directly involved in exercise need more oxygen and, therefore, require more blood flow. The skin receives more blood to help regulate body temperature and reduce body heat through the evaporation of sweat.

Metabolism

Metabolism is the body's process of converting food into energy through numerous chemical reactions (32). During an aerobic dance workout, as the muscles' need for oxygen increases, more energy is expended, which increases the metabolic rate (how rapidly the body uses its energy stores). Increased metabolic rate allows the body to use more energy—represented by calories—both during the workout and for approximately 1 to 2 hours after the workout.

BENEFITS OF AEROBICS

As you become regularly involved in an aerobic dance program, you can look forward to experiencing many of the benefits that accompany aerobic training. From the start of a new conditioning program, it will take approximately 8 to 10 weeks until changes (the training effect) will become apparent. Generally, the following changes in the body may be anticipated.

Cardiovascular Changes

With regular participation in aerobic exercise, the size of the ventricular cavity of the heart will increase slightly. This increase in the volume of the heart will in turn increase the stroke volume—the amount of blood ejected from the heart with each beat. An increase in stroke volume will increase the cardiac output—the amount of blood ejected from the heart each minute. All these changes will put less demand on the heart, as more blood will be ejected with each beat. This change decreases the resting heart rate (see Chapter 3) because the same amount of blood is ejected from the heart with fewer beats, placing less demand on the heart and thus increasing cardiac efficiency. Aerobic training also enhances the capillarization of the skeletal muscles by increasing the amount of oxygen and nutrients that can reach the muscles, which also contributes to improved cardiac efficiency.

With aerobic training, the level of **hemoglobin,** a protein cell present in the blood, increases. These cells carry the oxygen through the bloodstream and into the muscles, where ATP is then resynthesized and muscle contraction occurs. Larger amounts of hemoglobin cells will facilitate the delivery of oxygen to the working muscles and make muscular contraction easier. The exercising muscles' ability to extract the oxygen from the hemoglobin and then use it for contraction will also improve with regular aerobic exercise.

A final circulatory benefit that occurs with regular aerobic exercise is an increase of blood volume. With more blood available, once again more oxygen can be supplied to the muscle cell.

Respiratory Changes

As the depth of breathing increases with aerobic exercise, the respiratory muscles involved become more conditioned. An increase in ventilation efficiency means that less air needs to be ventilated (inhaled) to consume the same amount of oxygen. Because of improved breathing efficiency, the rate and depth of breathing at rest will also improve. Once again, the trained body does not have to work as hard for the same results.

Metabolic Changes

Trained muscles oxidize relatively more fat than do untrained muscles. The mechanism responsible for this change in energy metabolism is not entirely understood, but it may involve a greater capacity of the fat-burning enzymes in trained muscles to oxidize fatty acids (38). With the body's increased ability to metabolize fat there is an increase in the carbohydrate reserve. A conservation of carbohydrates can extend your performance time and let you exercise longer and harder before you become exhausted (36).

Body Composition

Aerobic exercise helps decrease body fat because, with increased activity, the body derives its energy from its fat stores. Regular participation in an aerobic training program generally reduces total body mass and fat weight; lean body weight may remain constant or increase (3).

Cardiac Risk

There are three primary risk factors associated with coronary heart disease:

1. Hypertension (high blood pressure)
2. High cholesterol levels
3. Cigarette smoking

There are also secondary risk factors:

1. Heredity
2. Sex (males are more prone than women)
3. Age
4. Stress
5. Obesity

Although much scientific evidence supports the view that exercise improves our health and that people who exercise are less susceptible to coronary heart disease, exercise cannot conclusively be prescribed as a prevention against cardiac disease. But let's look at how exercise affects the risk factors, and then you can draw your own conclusion.

People with hypertension can benefit from an aerobic program since aerobic exercise has been shown to lower systolic blood pressure in the hypertensive individual (24). Recent research has also shown that regular aerobic exercise can lead to a decrease in total blood cholesterol levels. There are two types of cholesterol: HDLs (high density lipoproteins), which appear to be protective against coronary heart disease, and LDLs (low density lipoproteins), which appear to contribute to its onset. Exercise will increase the HDLs in the bloodstream, whereas only diet can decrease the LDLs. With an increase of HDL cholesterol, the total cholesterol ratio is lowered, and that is positive for reducing the risk of coronary heart disease (24).

As discussed above, exercise can decrease obesity by reducing total body fat. As for the other risks, exercise obviously cannot alter age, sex, heredity, or the risks of cigarette smoking. (However, cigarette smoking can negatively affect exercise by impeding the hemoglobin's ability to carry oxygen to the blood.) It's true some things cannot be changed, but exercise can certainly delay the inevitable!

Psychological Benefits

For centuries, philosophers have discoursed about the concept of the total person: an individual who has a balanced relationship between mind and body. Health professionals advocate that involvement in regular physical exercise enhances the psychological well-being of a participant by reducing tension and stress, improving sleep habits, and increasing self-esteem and feelings of vitality. Unfortunately, there is not enough scientific evidence to support these beliefs in psychological benefits. However, one premise does remain true: People involved in a regular aerobic exercise program generally feel much better.

Benefits from Aerobic Exercise

Increase in heart volume
Increase in stroke volume
Increase in cardiac output
Increase in capillarization
Increase in blood volume
Increase in hemoglobin levels
Increase in ventilatory efficiency
Increase in muscles' ability to oxidize fat
Increase in metabolism
Possible increase in lean body mass

Decrease in resting heart rate
Decrease in exercise or target heart rate
Decrease in rate and depth of breathing at rest
Decrease in body fat
Decrease in blood pressure for the hypertensive
    individual

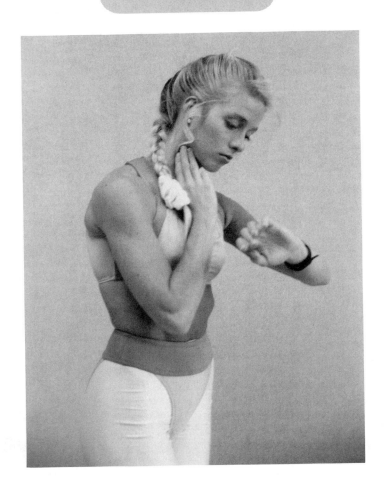

What the Heart Rate Tells Us

Chapter

3

The heart rate is the most readily obtainable measure of cardiorespiratory response to exercise. Because the heart rate is directly proportional to the intensity of exercise performed, it tells us whether we are working too hard or not hard enough. The pulse indicates the heartbeat and is counted in beats per minute. You can take your pulse at several different points on your body: the radial artery (at the base of your thumb on either arm), the carotid artery in your neck (on each side of your voice box), or at the temple in front of each ear (see Figure 3–1).

When monitoring your pulse, apply light pressure against the spot, using your first three fingers. Never use your thumb when monitoring your pulse because it has a pulse of its own and can give an inaccurate count.

When determining the exercise pulse, count each beat for 6 seconds and multiply the number by 10, or count for 10 seconds and multiply the number by 6. The negative aspect of the 6-count pulse is that a 1-count error will make a big difference in the beats per minute, whereas the negative aspect of the 10-second pulse is the difficulty of multiplying by 6. Determining the count for a short period is necessary because, when exercising, the pulse drops quickly; thus a longer pulse count would produce a less accurate measure. Whatever pulse technique you use, the most important aspect is to be consistent and to begin counting as soon as possible. Some people recommend starting the count with zero as opposed to one. Again, there is no critical difference between the two approaches. The main thing is to be con-

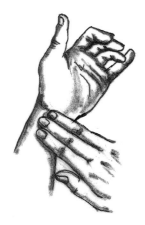

a. Radial artery

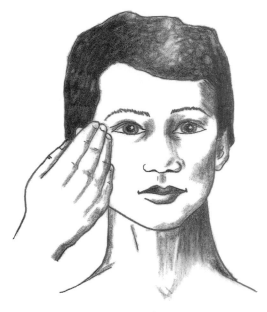

c. Temple

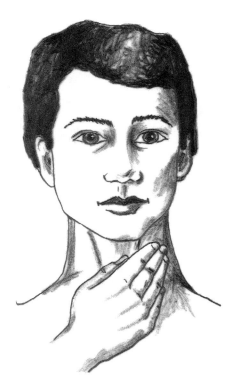

b. Carotid artery

Figure 3–1 *Sites to monitor your pulse.*

sistent with your technique so that changes can be accurately monitored. With practice, you will get a consistently reliable measure. In an aerobic dance program, it is important to know your resting heart rate and how to calculate your maximum, target, and recovery heart rates.

RESTING HEART RATE

You should take your **resting heart rate** when you first awake in the morning. At this time, only basal metabolic demands have been made on the heart and external stimuli have had no opportunity to affect the resting heart rate. In a comfortable, lying-down position, monitor your pulse for 30 seconds and multiply the number by 2. Unlike the exercise pulse, the resting pulse does not drop quickly, so a short pulse-taking time is unnecessary.

Typically, after a period of 6 to 8 weeks of aerobic exercise training, the resting heart rate will be lowered (20). Medical textbooks state that the average resting heart rate is 72 beats per minute. Highly trained athletes may have a resting heart rate of 40 beats per minute or lower. The slower

Track Your Resting Heart Rate

N A M E _____

Procedure: Determine your resting heart rate for 30 (multiply this number by 2) or 60 seconds when you first wake up after a full sleep. Lightly press your first three fingers on the radial artery, the carotid artery, or the temple.

Initial Assessment

Resting pulse _____   Date _____

8-Week Assessment

Resting pulse _____   Date _____

16-Week Assessment

Resting pulse _____   Date _____

Karvonen's Formula for Determining Target Heart Rate

Method	**Example 1**	**Example 2**
	A 20-year-old with a resting heart rate (RHR) of 80 beats per minute	A 40-year-old with a resting heart rate (RHR) of 80 beats per minute

STEP 1

Estimate your maximum heart rate by subtracting your age from 220.	220 − 20 200 maximum heart rate	220 − 40 180 maximum heart rate

STEP 2

Subtract your resting heart rate from your maximum heart rate.	200 maximum heart rate − 80 RHR 120	180 maximum heart rate − 80 RHR 100

STEP 3

Multiply the answer from step 2 by .6.	120 × .6 = 72	100 × .6 = 60
Multiply the answer from step 2 by .85.	120 × .85 = 102	100 × .85 = 85

STEP 4

To each figure in step 3, add your resting heart rate.	72 + 80 = 152 102 + 80 = 182	60 + 80 = 140 85 + 80 = 165

STEP 5

The range between these two sums is your target heart rate zone to use while exercising.	Target heart rate zone = 152−182 beats per minute	Target heart rate zone = 140−165 beats per minute

resting heart rate means that the heart does not have to beat as often to supply the body with blood and the heart has more rest between beats. You should monitor your resting heart rate after the first 8 weeks of training to evaluate any changes. Use the chart on page 19 to record your resting heart rate over a 16-week period.

Although regular aerobic training programs can reduce the resting heart rate, the following factors can also affect it:

Age: Resting heart rate generally increases with age.

Gender: Resting heart rate is generally higher in women.

Athletic training: Highly trained athletes usually have a lower resting heart rate.

Heredity: If there is a history of low or high resting heart rates within your family, you may inherit that trait.

Emotional stress: Intense emotional states can increase the resting heart rate.

Body temperature: When the body temperature is lower, the resting heart rate is lower. As the body temperature rises, it increases.

Age-Adjusted Target Heart Rate Chart for 60 to 85 Percent of Maximal Heart Rate

Age	Maximum Heart Rate	60%	85%
20	200	120	170
25	195	117	166
30	190	114	162
35	185	111	157
40	180	108	153
45	175	105	149
50	170	102	145
55	165	99	140
60	160	96	136
65	155	93	132
70	150	90	128

Smoking: Smoking even one cigarette increases the resting heart rate.

Caffeine: Caffeine intake increases the resting heart rate.

Physical illnesses: Colds, flus, and such increase the resting heart rate.

Birth control pills and other medications: These can increase the resting heart rate.

TARGET HEART RATE

When you are exercising to achieve a training effect, your heart must work hard enough to affect your aerobic capacity, but not so hard that you become fatigued. You should attempt to exercise *not* at your maximum heart rate, which is the highest heart rate you can attain and one that is impossible and even dangerous to sustain, but at your **target,** or exercise, **heart rate.**

However, you do need to know your maximum heart rate so that you can determine your target heart rate. You can predict your maximum heart rate by using this formula (25).

Maximum heart rate = 220 − your age

This predicted value varies among people of the same age group. However, the value is accurate enough for estimating your target heart rate.

Most experts agree that, for positive changes to occur in the cardiovascular system, exercise must be performed at an intensity high enough to increase the heart rate to about 70 percent of its maximum. Although no definite evidence is available, the upper limit for training intensity is thought to be about 85 percent of the maximum. For people in relatively poor condition, the training threshold may be closer to 60 percent of their maximum heart rate (38). The upper and lower limits depend a great deal on an individual's initial capacity and state of training.

In 1957, M. J. Karvonen, a Finnish researcher, found from a study of young men that, for appreciable gains in cardiorespiratory fitness to occur, during exercise the heart rate must be raised by a minimum of 60 percent of the difference between the maximum heart rate and the resting heart rate (38):

Target heart rate = resting heart rate
+ .60(maximum heart rate − resting heart rate)

Since Karvonen's findings, an increase in heart rate equal to between 60 and 85 percent of the maximum heart rate has been established as a safe and reasonable intensity. Two examples of how to calculate target heart rate with Karvonen's formula are illustrated in the table on page 20. A complete age-adjusted chart is also included above.

It is important that you check your heart rate at various intervals during the aerobic workout. Since heart rate reflects the level of stress on the

Borg Scale for Perceived Exertion*

Heart Rate Expected (for 20-year-old)	Perceived Exertion Rating	Description
60	6	
70	7	Very very light
80	8	
90	9	Very light
100	10	
110	11	Fairly light
120	12	
130	13	Somewhat hard
140	14	
150	15	Hard
160	16	
170	17	Very hard
180	18	
190	19	Very very hard
200	20	

* When using this scale, the subject is asked to identify by the number listed how he or she perceives the work.

Reprinted with permission from Borg, G.: Subjective effort in relation to physical performance and working capacity. In *Psychology: From Research to Practice,* edited by H. L. Pick, 333–61. New York: Plenum, 1978.

body, as long as you stay within the bounds of your target zone, you will be exercising safely. Beginners should continually check their pulse so that they do not exceed the high limits of the target zone; exceeding the upper limits brings on early fatigue and could discourage future aerobic activity by causing early burnout.

As the aerobic capacity of your cardiovascular system increases, work will become easier. You will therefore have to increase the intensity of your activities to work at the appropriate target heart rate.

Other Techniques for Measuring Intensity

The pulse is not always the most accurate method for measuring intensity because of individual variability. Some people may exceed their target heart rate zone yet feel fine, while other individuals may feel unable to keep pace with the workout although their pulse is below the target heart rate zone. Because of these variations, intensity can be monitored in other ways.

The Talk Test

The **talk test** merely means that you are able to carry on a conversation while you are exercising. If you are breathing so heavily that you cannot talk, then the intensity is too great. On the other hand, if you can sing a song, you are probably not working hard enough. Check your ability to talk frequently during the class, even if it is just to count along with the instructor!

Perceived Exertion

A **perceived exertion** scale was formalized by a man named Borg in 1982. The Borg Scale (see above) identifies the quantitative feelings of fatigue and is based on the heart rate of a 20-year-old. Subjects are asked to identify how they are feeling on a scale of 6–20. When using this scale, the level most appropriate for aerobic exercise is a range of 13–17. In Borg's terms, this is identified as "somewhat hard" to "very hard." (Beginners have a harder time perceiving their level of exertion, but as you learn the feelings of your body, this scale can be as relevant a measure of intensity as the heart rate.)

RECOVERY HEART RATE

Your **recovery heart rate,** which you should take 1 minute after you stop exercising, indicates how quickly you have recovered from an exercise session. Physically fit persons generally recover more rapidly because their cardiovascular systems are more efficient and adapt more quickly to the imposed demands.

The recovery heart rate really has two decreasing phases: the first minute after exercise, during which the heart rate drops sharply, and the *resting plateau,* during which the heart rate gradually decreases. The resting plateau may last as much as 1 hour after exercise. Five minutes following exercise, the heart rate should not exceed 120 beats per minute. After 10 minutes, the heart rate should be below 100 beats per minute. The heart rate should return to its preexercise rate approximately 30 minutes after the exercise session. However, the initial sharp drop in the heart rate that occurs 1 minute after the exercise is the most meaningful indicator of fitness. To determine your rate of recovery, use the following formula:

Recovery heart rate = (exercise heart rate − recovery heart rate after 1 minute) ÷ 10

Monitor your exercise pulse immediately at the end of your workout. Exactly 1 minute after the exercise, take your pulse again. Subtract the 1-minute recovery rate from the exercise heart rate and divide this figure by 10. The higher the number for the recovery rate, the more quickly your heart has recovered from the exercise. Use the following table to evaluate your recovery rate:

Number	*Condition*
Less than 2	Poor
2 to 3	Fair
3 to 4	Good
4 to 6	Excellent
Above 6	Outstanding

The recovery heart rate also measures the intensity of the workout. Very little drop in the 1-minute pulse would indicate that you were probably working too hard and your body was having a difficult time recuperating.

Your heart rate is your best indicator for determining your proper exercise intensity. Take your pulse often throughout the workout, until you learn what your body needs to sustain your target heart rate. Remember, increase the intensity of your exercise if you are not yet in your target range; decrease the intensity if the target rate is too high. Monitor your resting heart rate periodically to evaluate the effects of your aerobic training program. Generally, a lower resting heart rate means a healthier heart.

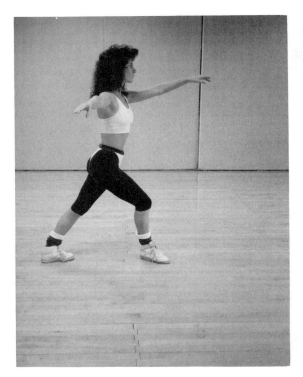
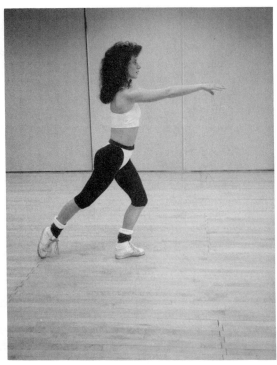

Take Care
of Your Body

Chapter

4

Before embarking on your first aerobic dance class, you should have some knowledge of injury prevention and care. No one cares more about your body than you do, so it is essential that you learn to take the best care of it. After all, it has to last you a lifetime! Involvement in a sport or recreational activity is not without risk of injury. However, aerobic dance, or any exercise program, is safe if you perform exercises with careful attention to proper technique and take certain precautions. You should recognize and follow the simple guidelines discussed in this chapter.

SELF-ASSESSMENT

The first phase of injury prevention involves self-assessment. Evaluate your readiness to begin an aerobic exercise program. If you are not sure you have the strength or stamina, discuss your doubts with the aerobics instructor or your doctor. Ask for an exercise program that will help build your strength slowly and safely.

FOLLOW YOUR FEELINGS

Do not force yourself to exercise when you are not feeling up to it; on the other hand, do not give in to every little excuse for avoiding your exercise class. A part of all of us would rather sit and relax. Learn to evaluate when to push yourself and when to go easy.

PAIN—A FRIENDLY SIGNAL

Pain is part of your body's language; it tells you when something is wrong. When you have pain, do not ignore it—investigate it. If your discomfort is beyond normal muscle soreness and does not go away or is recurring, seek professional evaluation and diagnosis.

SORENESS

Usually the most common ailment of the aerobics dancer is muscle soreness. When you begin an activity to which your body is not accustomed, you can expect a slight feeling of soreness. There are two different types of soreness. *General* or *acute soreness* occurs during or immediately after an exercise session and disappears in 3 to 4 hours. Acute soreness is thought to be induced by an inadequate blood flow to the exercising muscles (*ischemia*). This condition causes lactic acid and potassium end products to accumulate; this accumulation eventually stimulates pain receptors. When there is adequate blood flow to the active muscles, these end products are diffused and soreness diminishes.

The second type of soreness is *delayed muscle soreness,* which increases for 2 to 3 days following exercise and then diminishes until it disappears completely after 7 days. The four popular theories about the etiology of delayed muscle soreness are lactic acid accumulation, muscle spasms, torn muscle tissues, and damaged connective tissues.

The degree of delayed muscle soreness is related to the type of muscular contractions. During eccentric contractions, a muscle contracts as it lengthens. During concentric contractions, a muscle shortens as it contracts. Maximum soreness seems to be related to eccentric contractions (26).

You can help prevent some soreness by:

1. Warming up properly
2. Avoiding bouncing-type (ballistic) stretching
3. Progressing slowly into your aerobic dance program
4. Cooling down properly with adequate stretching

Expect some soreness if you have been inactive before starting your exercise program. Use sensible judgment regarding your body. Do not stop exercising merely because you are a little sore; the soreness will only recur later when you attempt another exercise program.

R-I-C-E: THE RECIPE FOR FIRST AID

Every athlete faces the risk of injury, and the aerobic dancer is no exception. Some athletic injuries merely require self-care treatment. However, other injuries require proper first aid treatment or, depending on their severity, professional diagnosis and treatment. Apply first aid as soon as you incur an injury. Immediate treatment quickens the healing process. A simple way to remember the first aid treatment is to keep in mind the initials R-I-C-E:

Rest
Ice
Compression
Elevation

Rest: Stop using the injured area as soon as you experience pain.

Ice: Ice reduces swelling and alleviates pain. Apply ice immediately to the injured area for 15 to 20 minutes several times a day for the first 24 hours after the injury has occurred. Let the injured body part regain its normal body temperature between icings.

Compression: Firmly wrap the injured body part with an elastic or compression bandage between icings. (A change in color or sensation in the extremities may mean the bandage is wrapped too tightly.)

Elevation: Raise the injured part above heart level to decrease the blood supply to the injured area.

You must let an injury heal completely before resuming activity. Once the injury has healed, reinitiate your aerobic dance training *slowly* so there will be no reinjury.

SELF-CARE INJURIES

The following injuries may require first aid treatment. If the injury does not heal with first aid treatment, consult a physician.

Stitch Pain

A pain in the side from running is called a *stitch pain,* which is the result of a spasm in the diaphragm. A stitch pain usually occurs when too much has been demanded from the diaphragm without proper preparation, that is, a proper warm-up. A stitch pain may also be due to a lack of oxygen and/or a buildup of carbon dioxide from poor rhythmical breathing. Although many instructors advise running through a stitch pain, this is *not* recommended because more muscle fibers of the diaphragm may become involved and thus increase the strain on the diaphragm.

There are two ways to get rid of a side stitch: bend over in the direction of the stitch or merely walk. If the spasm releases, gradually increase your speed from a jog to a full run. If the stitch pain persists or returns, *stop!*

Blister

A *blister,* caused by friction, is an escape of tissue fluid from beneath the skin's surface. You should not pop or drain a blister unless it interferes with your daily activity to the point where it absolutely has to be drained. If this is the case, clean the area affected with antiseptic. Then lance the blister with a sterile needle at several points and forcibly drain it. As the blister dries, leave the skin on for protection until the area of the blister forms "new" skin; then clip away the dead skin. You can prevent most blisters by taking sensible care of your feet and wearing properly fitting footwear.

Cramp

A *cramp* is a painful spasmodic muscle contraction. Muscle cramps commonly occur in the back of the lower leg (calf), the back of the upper leg (hamstring muscle group), and the front of the upper leg (quadriceps muscle group). Cramps are related to fatigue; muscle tightness; or fluid, salt, and potassium imbalance (19). To relieve the pain, gently stretch and/or massage the cramped muscle area. Since muscle cramps can be caused by a fluid and mineral imbalance from profuse sweating, drink water freely and increase your potassium intake naturally with foods such as tomatoes, bananas, and orange juice.

Muscle Strain

One type of muscle strain is the muscle pull, or damage to the muscle tissue. Scar tissue forms in the damaged area, and—because scar tissue is not as resilient as muscle tissue—you feel the effect of the pull for a long time. Another type of muscle strain involves the tissue around the muscle. The tendons, for example—the tissues that attach muscles to bones—often sustain strains. The blood supply to muscle-surrounding tissues is smaller than to the muscles; therefore, strains in these tissues take longer to heal than muscle pulls.

If you strain a muscle, apply ice as an immediate first aid treatment. Rest the injured area. Healing is affected by many factors—age, physical condition, and so on—so citing an "average" healing time could be misleading. If the condition of your strain does not improve in what you consider a reasonable time, consult a doctor.

INJURIES NEEDING PROFESSIONAL ATTENTION

More serious injuries that can be incurred from repeated jogging, jumping, and landing in an aerobic dance class are now described. These injuries usually require medical attention.

Shinsplints

Pain over the anterior aspect of the lower leg is generally called *shinsplints.* Shinsplints usually result from overuse of the muscle-tendon units. The major muscles of the lower leg are contained within fascia (tissue) envelopes. If there is swelling in the muscles, the arterial inflow and venous outflow to the muscles of that compartment can be impaired, causing a slow, activity-related pain in the involved compartment (11).

Several factors contribute to the development of shinsplints. One factor is an involuntary collapsing of the arch of the foot, which causes the muscles of the medial longitudinal arch, rather than its ligaments, to support the bones of the arch. Since the ligaments are intended to be the primary supporters, when the muscles are forced to assume that role, they become overfatigued, irritated, and inflamed.

Another factor is an imbalance of muscular strength on the front (anterior) and the back (posterior) aspect of the shinbone (the tibia) (35). Jogging or jumping on hard surfaces, improper landings from jumps, and improper shoes are also factors contributing to the development of shinsplints.

Plantar Fascitis

Plantar fascitis is a direct injury or strain of the plantar fascia, the ligamentous support of the arch of the foot. The injury causes chronic pain and inflames the foot, in particular, the heel. A radiating discomfort may also affect the longitudinal arch. Another cause of plantar fascitis is overuse by putting too much stress on the feet in relation to the amount of conditioning training and preparation.

Achilles Tendinitis

Inflammation of the Achilles tendon, the tendon of the heel, is common to running sports. *Achilles tendinitis* is often the result of a single episode of overuse. However, it can often be the result of a muscle imbalance of the lower leg.

Sprain

More serious than a strain, a *sprain* is a sudden or violent twisting or wrenching of a joint, causing the ligaments to stretch or tear and often the blood vessels to rupture, with hemorrhage into the surrounding tissues. Symptoms of a sprain are swelling, inflammation, point tenderness, and discoloration. Ankle sprains are the most common in aerobic dance. The most frequent is the *inversion sprain,* which results from unstable landings (5). The ligaments on the outside of the ankle joint are the weakest in the ankle and are most susceptible to injury incurred by rolling over on the outside of the ankle.

Chondromalacia Patella (Runner's Knee)

Aerobic dancers may experience a vague pain in the knees when running, leaping, or stair stepping (or walking or running up and down stairs). This pain is characteristic of *chondromalacia patella,* or runner's knee—an erosion of the cartilage covering the underside of the kneecap, or patella. Internal factors that affect chondromalacia are anatomical malalignment of the lower extremities:

Discrepancy in leg length
Abnormality in rotation of the hips
Bowlegs
Knock-knees
Flatfeet
Musculature imbalance

The following external factors can also promote the problem:

Training errors, including abrupt changes in intensity, duration, or frequency
Improper footwear
Bad running surfaces (3); avoid dancing on cement floors

Patellar Tendinitis (Jumper's Knee)

Repetitive jumping and landing activities can produce small scars in the patellar tendon, causing pain, tenderness, and inflammation directly below the kneecap. Often an aching in the knees apparent at the beginning of a workout disappears after warm-up. However, pain recurs when activity ceases. In a worsened condition, pain continues throughout a workout, and pressing on the tendon itself causes pain.

Stress Fracture

A *stress fracture* is a small fracture caused by repetitive jogging, jumping, and landing. In most cases, it occurs in the shins or the ball of the foot, involving one or both of the small sesamoid bones located in this area of the foot. The injury causes chronic pain and swelling.

SUMMARY

Any sort of injury can take time away from your aerobic training program. Use proper precautions and common sense in initiating your training. If you are injured, remember the simple steps of first aid treatment: rest, ice, compression, and elevation; apply the treatment immediately after injury occurs. Seek medical advice for injuries that persist.

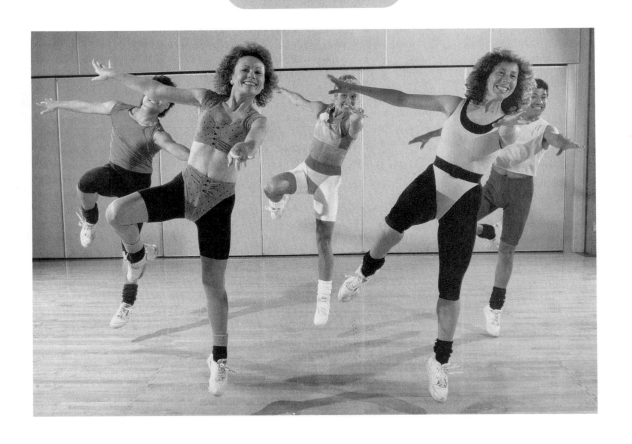

What to Expect in an Aerobic Dance Class

Chapter

5

The aerobic dance class is a successful combination of exercise, fitness, and fun. If you are enrolling in an aerobic dance class for the first time, you need to know what to expect from the class and what is expected of you in the class. This chapter describes the basic structure of an aerobic dance class and outlines the importance of regular attendance and participation, the need for individualized pacing, and what to wear.

MEDICAL CONSIDERATIONS

Before embarking on an aerobic dance program, you may want to consider a medical evaluation of your current health status. If you have been following a regular exercise program, an aerobic dance class should pose no physical problems.

However, if you have a serious medical problem and are concerned about the possible effects of increased physical activity, check with your doctor. Your doctor will help you decide whether or not you can safely participate in an aerobic dance class. Students should complete the chart on the next page for the instructor's use.

STRUCTURE OF AN AEROBIC DANCE CLASS

Aerobic dance combines walking and jogging with jumps, hops, kicks, and lunges as well as basic calisthenics to improve muscular strength, endurance, and flexibility. Aerobic dance also develops coordination and rhythm by combining simple dance movements into choreographed routines.

Aerobic Student Health History

N A M E _____ **A G E** _____ **D A T E** _____

C L A S S _____ **S E C T I O N** _____

1. Do you have any of the following conditions?

   _____ Diabetes   _____ Epilepsy

   _____ Hypertension   _____ Asthma

2. Have you had any of the following within the past 2 years?

   _____ Heart attack

   _____ Stroke

   _____ Heart surgery

   _____ General major surgery   Please specify _____

3. Do you smoke? Yes _____   No _____

   Cigarettes per day _____   Cigars _____   Pipe _____

4. Are you currently taking any medication? Yes _____   No _____

   Please specify _____

5. Are you currently under a doctor's care? Yes _____   No _____

   Reason _____

6. Do you have any handicaps or current injuries that limit your physical activity?

   Yes _____   No _____

   Please specify _____

   _____

7. Date of last physical examination _____

8. Additional information _____

   _____

The routines should be fun and easy to perform with a variety of musical selections. Although all instructors have their own personal lesson formats, the following structure is typical of an aerobic dance class.

WARM-UP

The warm-up eases the body from a resting state into one of activity. This phase of the class is designed to increase the heart rate and the body's core temperature. The warm-up, generally lasting 5 to 10 minutes, prepares the body for the movements to be performed in the aerobic conditioning phase of the lesson.

The warm-up usually consists of three phases. The first phase is a series of loosening, isolation exercises for the neck, shoulders, trunk and hips, knees, and ankles. The second phase involves an active warm-up of controlled, full-body movements to achieve an elevation in body temperature. During the third phase, simple stretches specifically for the shoulders, spine, quadriceps, hamstrings, calf muscles, and Achilles tendons are executed to enhance flexibility and reduce injury risk for the workout ahead.

LOW-IMPACT AEROBICS, OR FIRST-PHASE AEROBICS

Following the warm-up, the aerobic conditioning, or first, phase of the aerobic lesson begins with low-impact aerobic routines. These initial routines are of low to moderate intensity and incorporate full-body movements emphasizing large muscle groups. Routines move around the room in a variety of directional patterns in order to increase the heart rate and decrease impact. During this low-impact aerobic session, the heart rate and oxygen consumption gradually increase so that, by the end, the target heart rate zone is achieved.

PEAK AEROBICS

Depending on the lesson format and aerobic training requirements, the aerobic session continues by advancing to high-impact routines and/or more strenuous low-impact moves. All routines are designed to keep the heart rate within the target heart rate zone and can be modified to suit the individual's fitness level. The main emphasis is to "keep moving." Between dances, the pulse rate is often monitored, but even when monitoring their pulse, students maintain at least a walking pace. The entire aerobic phase lasts between 20 and 30 minutes.

AEROBIC COOL-DOWN

The aerobic cool-down follows the peak aerobic phase of the lesson and is generally a continuation of aerobic dance movements performed at a lower intensity and/or a slowing down of locomotor movements to a walking pace. Basically, the aerobic cool-down is a tapering of exercise in order to return the pulse to below the target heart rate zone. Stretches specifically for the quadriceps, hamstrings, calf muscles, and Achilles tendons can also be performed at the end of this cool-down phase.

BODY TONING AND CONDITIONING

Body toning and conditioning exercises may follow either the warm-up or the aerobic routines. This exercise period lasts 5 to 20 minutes and stresses muscular strength and flexibility. The exercises concentrate on increasing endurance and strengthening and toning the muscles of the arms, abdomen, buttocks, and thighs, with attention to body alignment and good exercise technique.

FLEXIBILITY COOL-DOWN

The warm-up prepares the body for activity; the flexibility cool-down prepares the body for rest. This phase, lasting 5 to 10 minutes, involves a series of slow stretches and movements that improve flexibility and gradually slow down the body so that the exercise period does not end abruptly. It is most important at this time to achieve maximum flexibility while the muscles are still warm. Static stretching helps to maintain and/or increase flexibility and prevent muscle soreness.

RELAXATION

Rest is the relaxation phase of the exercise cycle. Being able to relax is as important to the body as being able to successfully withstand imposed physical demands. The relaxation phase of the aerobic dance lesson is 5 to 10 minutes long. It incorporates breathing techniques and/or active or passive relaxation activities (see Chapter 13).

REGULAR ATTENDANCE

To achieve fitness benefits from an aerobic dance program, you must attend class (or participate in aerobic activity) at least three times a week for a minimum of 20 minutes. These classes should be evenly distributed throughout the week, with a maximum of two days' rest between classes. If you must miss a class, substitute a jog, quick walk, or another aerobic activity within the week.

If you are ill or unable to exercise over a certain length of time, it is important to gradually work your way back to your former level of activity. It may take you three or more classes after an illness to perform with the same energy you expended prior to your absence. With regular participation, you can maintain and improve fitness levels.

INDIVIDUAL PACE

We have all heard the fitness axioms "Train, don't strain" and "No pain, no gain." Somewhere between these two ideas is a middle ground that provides the safest and most productive workout pace. You are not competing with anyone but yourself in aerobic dance, so it is important to work at your own level; set the pace that is most beneficial for your own body. Keep breathing easily, and never hold your breath. If you can carry on a conversation when performing aerobic dance, you are working at the correct pace.

In aerobic dance, the heartbeat is regularly monitored to help establish a pace that will push a person to achieve but not overexert. Aerobic dance routines are choreographed so that, depending on the individual fitness level, sections of routines allow students to participate at their own desired impact or intensity level.

SIGNS OF OVERTRAINING

In Chapter 3 we discussed measuring intensity as an important tool for working correctly and effectively in class. There are times though when students can get carried away with the enthusiasm of the class and forget to pay attention to their heart rate or perceived exertion. If this extends for much of the class period, the following signs of *acute* overtraining may occur during the workout:

1. Rapid breathing and inability to talk
2. Profuse sweating
3. Extreme redness in the face
4. Inability to keep up with the basic class movements
5. Dizziness or light-headedness

If any of these symptoms should occur, you should immediately slow down your activity and decrease the intensity of the moves.

Lower the intensity of aerobic dance movements by:

1. Decreasing the size or range of the movements
2. Lessening the use of the arms or lowering the arm movements to below heart level
3. Slowing down the movements

If you stay within your appropriate exercise range, you will maintain a positive attitude toward exercise: Workout, *don't* burnout!

There are also signs of overtraining that occur after the workout is over. These are termed *chronic* signs of overtraining. If you notice any of the following, a break from exercise or a reduction in intensity or duration might be appropriate:

Increase in resting heart rate
Chronic fatigue
Lack of motivation
Inability to relax
Extreme muscle soreness and stiffness the day after a workout
Decrease in body weight when no effort to decrease weight is being made
Lowered general physical resistance, such as a continuous cold or headache
Loss of appetite

Constipation or diarrhea

Unexplained drop in athletic performance (23)

WHAT TO WEAR

Comfortable clothing that allows ease of movement is appropriate attire for aerobic dancing. Sweatsuits and jogging apparel provide layers that you can remove as your body temperature increases. Once your body is warm, simple jogging shorts and a T-shirt or dance leotard and tights are sufficient. Cotton is the best material for exercise wear because it absorbs perspiration. As cotton becomes damp, the air evaporates the moisture and cools your body.

The fashion industry has provided an assortment of specialty aerobic dance apparel. Overgarments that superficially heat the body include legwarmers, wool unitards and tights, and nylon rip pants, shorts, and tops. These clothing items should be worn only as overgarments or to warm up the body. A popular notion is that use of these items during a workout can lead to quick weight loss, but in truth you are only sweating off water—not fat! In warm weather you should wear the minimum amount of clothing so that you can sweat freely and let your cooling system work.

Support undergarments are important apparel in aerobic dance. Women should wear a bra that fits snugly and provides adequate support during the vigorous running and jumping movements in class. Men should wear athletic supporters or dance belts for adequate support during exercise activities.

Shoes

Foot Facts

Your foot is a complicated structure made up of 26 bones, 33 joints, and about 20 muscles that control movement. There are three basic foot types; your type of foot dictates the type of shoe you should wear for an aerobic dance class.

The ball of the *normal foot* rests on the ground regardless of whether or not the heel is lifted. The normal foot will fit most shoes as long as the heel

fits snugly and the shoe accommodates the width of the foot.

The *cavos foot* has a high arch and tends to absorb shock poorly. This type of foot needs a shoe with a firm counter (the stiff piece around the heel, usually of leather). Additionally, heel lifts may sometimes be necessary for the high-arch foot.

The *flatfoot* has a poor arch and has no rise to the top portion of the foot when viewed from the side. The flatfoot requires a very firm counter and a very firm midsole.

Shoe-Buying Tips

Shoes are the major monetary investment for an aerobic dance class and the most important item you wear to class. Most aerobic shoes today provide stability at the rear of the foot, where shock absorbency and stability are needed during exercise. As you look at the many models available, keep in mind your specific foot type and consider the following points as you compare shoes:

1. Leather is the best material for aerobic shoes because it breathes and molds to your foot. A hard leather gives better support than a soft leather, which stretches after a few wearings.
2. Lateral support straps (straps that cross the upper) provide foot stability. Straps that are close to the front of the shoe (closer to the toe) provide greater support.
3. The sole width should match the heel width. If the sole is too narrow, it will not provide enough stability for your foot during landing.
4. There should be an adequate longitudinal arch support.
5. The sole should be flexible at the ball of the foot with a flexible upper also available.
6. The toe box should be high enough so you can wiggle all your toes within the shoe.
7. There should be a padded heel collar.

In-store Shoe Test

Keep in mind the type of flooring on which you will be exercising and try to test your shoe on a surface in the store that most resembles the one in the class. If you aerobic dance on carpet, look for a shoe with a smooth tread, which will allow you

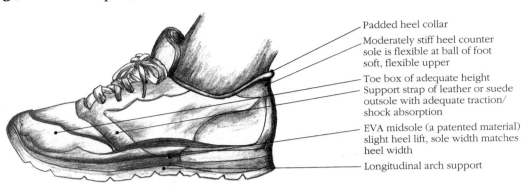

Padded heel collar
Moderately stiff heel counter
sole is flexible at ball of foot
soft, flexible upper
Toe box of adequate height
Support strap of leather or suede
outsole with adequate traction/
shock absorption
EVA midsole (a patented material)
slight heel lift, sole width matches
heel width
Longitudinal arch support

Diagram of an appropriate aerobic shoe

to perform twisting and turning movements more easily. If your workout surface is hard, look for shoes with shock-absorbent midsoles.

Try some aerobic dance moves and see how the shoe feels:

1. Roll forward on the balls of your feet. The shoe should bend at the same point where your foot bends. A lack of flexibility in the shoe may cause strain in the ball and/or arch of your foot.
2. Hop on one foot to test shock absorption.
3. Stand on one foot. Keep your foot in place as you twist your upper body and hop left and right. This will cause your supporting foot to roll inward and outward, testing shoe stability. You should feel balanced as you twist if the shoe is stable.
4. Stand on one foot and raise your heel so that you are on the ball of your foot. As in test 3, twist to test shoe stability.
5. Run in place and in various movement patterns. The shoe should feel snug, but you should be able to wiggle your toes (17).

As you test several pairs of shoes, select a pair that performs the best for you. For further care of your feet, remember to wear cotton socks with shoes to keep your feet dry and free of blisters. Use foot powder or foot spray if your feet perspire heavily.

(Besides proper footwear for preventing injury, the composition of the dance floor is extremely important and should be investigated when you are choosing a class. Cement covered with carpet is the worst flooring because it gives the illusion of being cushioned, yet cement is the hardest possible surface. Hardwood flooring is the best surface for aerobic dance.)

WHAT TO BRING TO CLASS

A few additional items may be useful in your aerobic dance class: floor mat, towel, sweatbands, and light weights.

Floor Mat

A mat provides padded support for your body as you do floor exercises. If mats are not available at the class, you can buy a lightweight mat at most athletic stores, in the athletic department at a major department store, or at a chain drugstore. Any mat that is easy to carry and has some padding is sufficient.

Towel

A towel is useful in class if you perspire heavily. You can also use a towel to cover your mat, which is especially advisable if the mat is plastic because the towel will help absorb the additional perspiration the plastic creates.

Sweatbands

If you do not have a towel, wear a sweatband around your head and wrists to collect perspiration. Elasticized cotton sweatbands are easy to slip on and off. You can also use a bandana rolled and tied around your head as a sweatband.

Light Weights and Resistance Bands

Light weights and resistance bands are used by many instructors as a means to create resistance during body toning exercises. These bands and weights are specifically designed for conditioning exercises and can be purchased from aerobic dance and fitness suppliers.

CHECKLIST FOR A SUCCESSFUL CLASS

1. Arrive at class 10 to 15 minutes early to give yourself time for pre-warm-up exercises.
2. Do not eat a heavy meal prior to class. Fruit, yogurt, dried fruit, or nuts are recommended preclass snacks.
3. Come to class in the appropriate dance attire.
4. Clear your mind of outside interference when you enter the classroom. Be prepared to fully concentrate on the lesson.
5. Find a space to stand where you can see and hear the teacher. Allow yourself plenty of room so you can move and stretch freely.
6. Be sensitive to any injuries you might have. Pay special attention to the injured area during pre-warm-up exercises as well as class activities.
7. Work at your correct heart rate so you can keep moving and get maximum benefits from the workout.
8. Do not compare yourself to others in the class. Listen to your body!
9. Do not be afraid to ask questions if you are unclear about a step or exercise.
10. Bring a container of water for an occasional drink to avoid dehydration.
11. Participate in aerobic dance to improve your fitness, your posture, and your knowledge of your body and to have a good time!

Now that you know what to expect in your aerobic dance class, it is time to get started. The last ingredients to bring to class are the enthusiasm for doing your best and the attitude that you will have a good time!

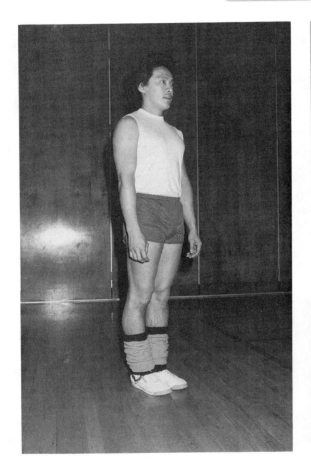
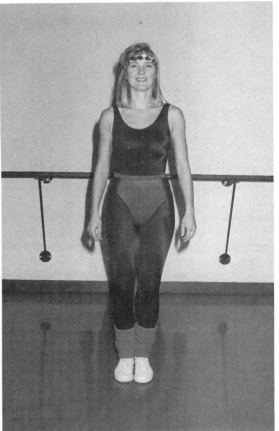

Posture Perfect—or Imperfect?

Chapter

There are several reasons why the aerobic dancer needs good posture: Good posture is the basis for effective movement patterns, it helps prevent injury, and aesthetically it creates the best body image. Correct skeletal alignment is also necessary to establish maximum balance and ease of movement. This chapter describes correct posture and body alignment and presents exercises to help you achieve correct posture.

POSTURE, PLACEMENT, AND ALIGNMENT

The key to achieving awareness of effective movement is understanding the differences between posture, placement, and alignment. **Posture** is the position of the body. **Placement** refers to weight carriage. You know from experience

that, without visibly changing your position, you can shift your weight from, say, the front of your foot to your heels. This weight shift is placement. Correct placement is critical for efficient and effective movement. **Alignment** is the relationship of the body segments to each other. A person may assume a posture correctly but be incorrectly placed and aligned.

Posture, placement, and alignment are the basics of movement. Of these three, alignment is the most fundamental because it defines the position of the body before movement begins. When the body is aligned, there is minimum strain on the muscles and ligaments attached to the weight-bearing joints. A misaligned aerobics dancer has a strong chance of becoming an injured dancer.

Correct alignment depends on a balanced relationship between the front (anterior) and the

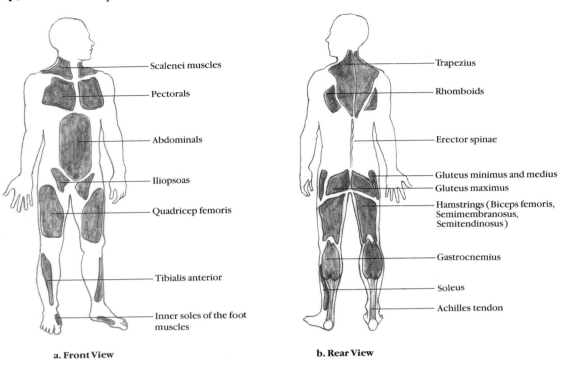

a. **Front View**   b. **Rear View**

Figure 6–1 *General location of postural muscles.*

back (posterior) postural muscles. Most of the large muscles in the body are involved with the body's maintenance of correct alignment. These muscles are classified as the *anteroposterior antigravity muscles* and are identified in Figure 6–1. The antigravity musculature helps the body adequately resist the pull of gravity so it can maintain an erect posture. These muscles must be well conditioned to withstand the stresses gravity imposes and to resist the skeletal framework's tendency to collapse with the force of gravity.

The downward pressure of gravity tends to make the skeletal framework misalign at three principal areas: the ankles, knees, and hips. To counteract this effect, the anteroposterior muscles must maintain a muscular tension balance. The muscles that maintain lower limb balance are the gastrocnemius and soleus at the ankle, the quadricep femoris at the knee, and the gluteus

maximus at the hip. The trunk is held erect by the erector spinae muscles running from the base of the skull to the sacrum. To balance the trunk's posterior aspect, the abdominals maintain the proper relationship between the rib cage and pelvis on the body's anterior aspect (22). An unbalanced relationship among these muscles will cause postural deviations.

ALIGNMENT REFERENCE POINTS

Basic body structure is, of course, determined by the skeleton. Figure 6–2 shows the major structural elements from the front. Figure 6–3 shows them from the back. Every individual's body structure is different, but there are visual guidelines for evaluating alignment. Figure 6–4 shows a side view of a body in correct alignment. The dotted line in the figure represents the line of

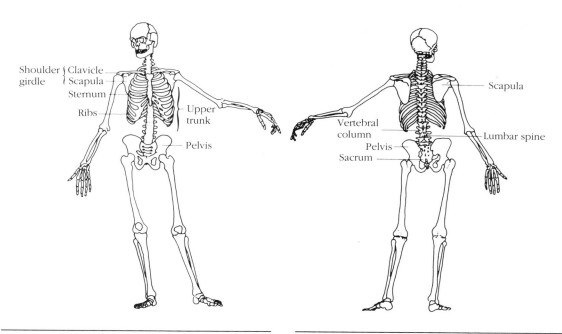

Figure 6–2 *Important skeletal structures, front view.*

Figure 6–3 *Important skeletal structures, rear view.*

gravity, which pulls straight down on the body. In a correctly aligned body, the line passes through the specific points shown in the figure. These points, called *alignment reference points,* are

    The top of the ear
    The middle of the shoulder girdle
    The center of the hip
    The back of the kneecap
    The front of the anklebone

Figure 6–4 shows that the spine is naturally curved. Figure 6–5 shows the curves more clearly. The two most evident curves are in the neck and lower back. These curves absorb the shock of normal movement and protect the upper body from jarring. Do not try to eliminate or exaggerate the natural curves. The dangers of doing so range from postural deviation to serious nerve and organ damage.

Figure 6–6 shows a correctly aligned body from the back. The line of gravity passes through the following alignment reference points:

    The center of the head
    The midpoint of all vertebrae
    The cleft of the buttocks
    Midway between the heels

Now consider the correctly aligned body in detail, from head to toe.

HEAD AND NECK

The head, the heaviest body segment, rests on the neck, which is a small, flexible segment. The head should be carried directly atop the neck, not ahead or behind it. There should be a sense of the neck stretching away from the spine so that both the back and the front of the neck are long. With

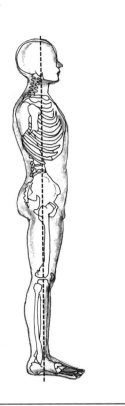

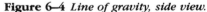

Figure 6–4 *Line of gravity, side view.*

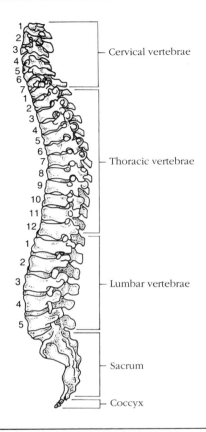

1
2
3   — Cervical vertebrae
4
5
6
7
1
2
3
4
5
6
7   — Thoracic vertebrae
8
9
10
11
12
1
2
3   — Lumbar vertebrae
4
5
      — Sacrum
      — Coccyx

Figure 6–5 *The spine, with its natural curves. (Adapted from Aerobic Dance—Exercise Instructor Manual* [San Diego: Idea Foundation, 1987] 41)

the head and neck in correct alignment, a vertical line can be drawn from the top of the ear to the middle of the shoulder girdle.

SHOULDER GIRDLE

The shoulder girdle—consisting of the clavicle in front and the scapula in back—should be directly above the rib cage. The shoulder girdle is attached to the trunk only at the sternum (breastbone), allowing it to move freely. The shoulders should not be pulled back or allowed to slump forward; they should point directly to the side so

that the chest is not collapsed and the shoulder blades are not pinched. The arms should hang freely in the sockets. The shoulders should be low enough and the neck "long" enough to maximize the distance between the shoulders and the ears.

RIB CAGE

The rib cage floats above the pelvis and is connected in back to the spinal column. The rib cage should be pulled in toward the spine and lifted upward from the pelvis to create a long-waisted appearance.

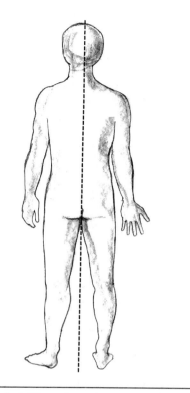

Figure 6–6 *Line of gravity, back view.*

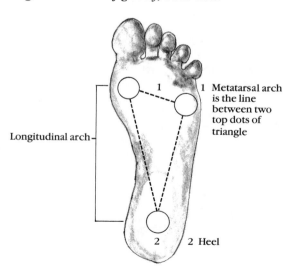

Figure 6–7 *Weight-bearing areas in the foot.*

PELVIS AND LOWER BACK

The pelvis is the keystone of the skeleton. The tilt of the pelvis affects the posture of the entire body and the distribution of the body's weight over the feet. To be correctly placed, the pelvis should be in a neutral position—neither tilted excessively forward nor backward—which lengthens the lumbar spine and shortens the abdominal muscles. Extreme forward or backward tilting of the pelvis can injure the lumbar spine and muscles of the lower back.

When the pelvis tilts forward, the lumbar area of the lower spine is forced to curve abnormally. The posterior discs located between the vertebrae are depressed, which results in lower back pain. When the pelvis is tilted backward, the natural lumbar curve is flattened. Anterior (forward) and posterior (backward) tilt can be rectified by proper conditioning of the vertebrae column and pelvic musculature.

KNEES

The knee position, which is affected by the placement of the pelvis, should be directly above and in line with the direction of the toes. In the standing position, the knees should be slightly relaxed. Hyperextension (a locking or pressing too far back) of the knees is a common error.

FEET

Although the pelvis is the keystone of the skeletal structure, the feet provide the main base of support. In a static position, the greatest support is achieved when the weight of the body is equally distributed over the metatarsal arch—the base of the big toe to the base of the small toe—and the heel (see Figure 6–7). All the toes should remain in contact with the floor to provide the widest possible base of support. In addition, the longitudinal arch should be well lifted to prevent the ankle from rolling inward.

ALIGNMENT EXERCISES

Exercises to help achieve correct body alignment follow. These exercises may be performed easily in 10 minutes and can serve as a pre-warm-up or as part of the stretch and relaxation segment at the end of class. It is recommended that they be performed daily, until correct alignment becomes a habit.

STARTING POSITION FOR ALIGNMENT EXERCISES

Lie on your back with your knees bent, soles of the feet flat on the ground, arms by the side of the body, and the palms of both hands flat on the floor. In this position, with the knees bent, the natural curve of the lower back is diminished somewhat to protect it from strain.

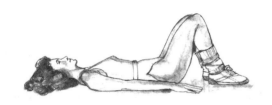

Starting position

ALIGNMENT OF THE NECK AND PELVIS

Assume the starting position and take deep breaths. As you exhale, allow the abdomen to contract. At the same time, attempt to lengthen the neck along the floor, pressing the chin slightly down. Hold this position, concentrating on the position of the neck, lower back, and abdomen. Repeat the exercise four times. Maintain the position of the abdomen, lower back, and neck throughout the remaining exercises.

ALIGNMENT OF THE SHOULDER GIRDLE

Assume the starting position and place both hands on the hipbones. Keeping your elbows in

contact with the floor, try to stretch to point the elbows toward the sides of the room. Hold for 10 seconds, then relax. Repeat this stretch four times. Although the movement of this exercise is slight, when executed properly, it will expand the back and the chest equally. Maintain this back and chest expansion throughout the remaining exercises.

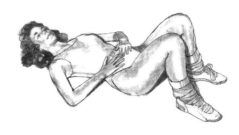

Shoulder girdle alignment, elbows touching floor

ALIGNMENT OF THE SHOULDER GIRDLE

Assume the starting position, with your hands placed on your hipbones. Isolate your shoulders by lifting them forward off the floor. Hold this position for 5 seconds. Relax and place your shoulders in contact with the floor. As this exercise is performed, attempt to create the greatest distance possible between your shoulders and ears. This will help to maintain the correct shoulder and neck alignment. Repeat the exercise four times.

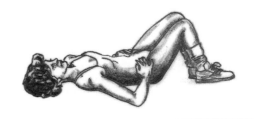

Shoulder girdle alignment, maintaining neck alignment

ALIGNMENT OF THE RIB CAGE

Assume the starting position, with your hands on your hipbones. Lift your rib cage off the floor to create an extreme arch in the back, keeping the shoulders planted firmly on the floor. Reverse the action, pressing the rib cage back against the floor, or further toward the spine. This position, with the rib cage pressed down, is correct alignment. Repeat the exercise four times, ending with the rib cage in its correct position against the floor.

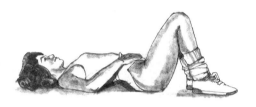

Rib cage alignment

After completing the last exercise, mentally review the correct alignment of the body parts:

Abdominal muscles contracted
Back and chest equally expanded, with elbows pointing to the side
Neck and ears stretching away from the spine and shoulders
Shoulders resting flat against the floor
Lower back in contact with the floor
Breathing full and easy

Come to a standing position.

ALIGNMENT IN A STANDING POSITION

Stand against a wall with your heels about 2 inches from the wall and your knees slightly bent. Assume the same body alignment you just experienced on the floor, keeping in mind the mental cues just outlined. Hold this position for a minimum of 20 seconds. Once you feel comfortable in this position, try to maintain this alignment while walking around the room.

LOWER BACK PAIN

Lower back pain is a problem many people experience. In this section we will outline the major causes of lower back pain and then describe exercises to help alleviate the pain or make it more manageable.

Causes of Lower Back Pain

There are many factors involved in lower back pain. Prolonged sitting—an occupational hazard built into many jobs—can create unnecessary tension in the lower back by causing the lumbar vertebral muscles to become shortened and thus inflexible and by encouraging weakened abdominal muscles. When a sudden stress is then placed on the back during exercise or when performing a daily task, the tightened muscles will strain and overstretch to accomplish the task and injury and pain may result.

Another factor contributing to lower back problems is incorrect posture. When the muscles are continually held in an imbalanced position, the lower back muscles excessively contract in order to keep the spine vertical. This will eventually cause lower back pain.

Faulty body mechanics, such as lifting heavy objects with the knees straight, is another way to put undue stress on the lower back. It is very important to bend the knees when lifting objects lower than the body. It is also important to keep the weight as close to the body as possible. The farther the weight is held away from the body, the more strain and possible injury can occur to the lower back.

Minimal physical activity, poor muscle tone, and excess weight, particularly in the abdomen, are other major factors that contribute to lower back pain. Regular exercise, with an emphasis on specific strength and flexibility exercises, will help alleviate these problems.

Weak abdominal muscles and inflexible muscles of the lower back are conditions that allow the pelvis to tilt forward, resulting in undue stress on lower back vertebrae. The following activities are important in helping to prevent lower back pain:

1. Perform strengthening exercises for the abdominals and gluteal muscles

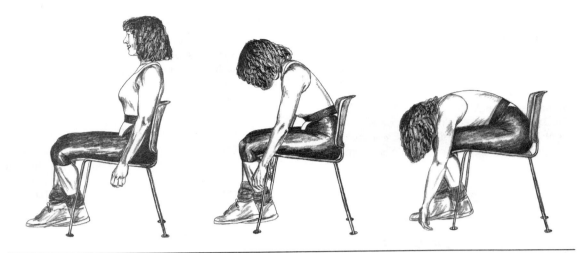

Lower back stretch

2. Perform flexibility exercises for the lower back, hamstring, and hip flexor muscles
3. Maintain good posture
4. Execute good exercise technique and body mechanics

Outlined below are specific exercises to help relieve muscular lower back pain.

Lower Back Exercises

Flexibility Exercises for the Lower Back Muscles, Hamstrings, and Hip Flexors

The *lower back muscles* are the muscles of the sacrum, connecting the vertebrae to the pelvis. They extend the lower back (arching backwards) and increase the curve of the lower back. For a healthy back, these muscles need flexibility.

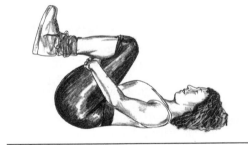

Double knee hold

LOWER BACK STRETCH

Sitting in a chair with your legs together or on the floor with your legs crossed, exhale and slowly bend forward one vertebra at a time. Relax in this position with your head as close to your knees as possible. Hold this position for 10 seconds and then slowly recover.

DOUBLE KNEE HOLD

Lying on your back, place your hands under your knees to keep pressure off the joints and bring both knees to your chest. Stretch your lower back by pulling gently on the lower leg, exhaling as you do this. Hold this position for several seconds.

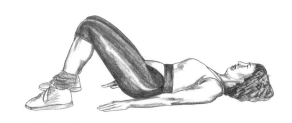

Pelvic tilt

PELVIC TILT

Lie on your back with your knees bent, feet flat on the floor, and hands at your side. Slowly contract the abdominal and buttocks muscles. The hips will lift slightly off the floor. Hold the contraction for 10 seconds and then release. Repeat this exercise 5 times.

Hip flexors are the muscles of the thighs (quadriceps) and the deep muscles of the pelvis (iliopsoas). They keep the pelvis in proper alignment. When they are tight, there is an extreme forward tilt of the pelvic girdle (swayback, or lordosis). See Chapter 7 for descriptions of the quadricep stretch and the runner lunge—a good stretch for the iliopsoas muscles.

The *hamstrings* are the muscles on the back of the thigh. They are a two-joint muscle that extends the hip and flexes the knee. When these muscles are inflexible, the curve in the lower back is increased, which causes lower back pain. It is very common for runners to have tight hamstrings. Hamstring stretches are found in Chapter 7.

Strengthening Exercises for the Gluteals and the Abdominals

The *gluteal muscles* are located in the buttocks. They are the hip extensors. Along with the muscles on the front of the hip, these muscles maintain proper alignment of the pelvis. When they are overly stretched, the pelvis will have an extreme forward tilt. Strengthening exercises for these muscles are described in Chapter 11 under exercises for the hips and buttocks.

The *abdominal muscles* also help to keep the pelvis in proper alignment. When these muscles are weak, the lower back muscles must overcompensate to keep the body erect. This causes lower back pain. Perform the abdominal exercises described in Chapter 11 to increase abdominal strength.

To totally alleviate lower back pain, the exercises recommended in this section should be performed on a daily basis. Even more important than performing the exercises, it is imperative to achieve an awareness of proper body alignment. When your body knows the correct placement of the pelvis, the lower back muscles will not be overtightened but will be in balance with the muscles on the front of the pelvis. When this correct placement becomes habitual, then the lower back will be free from pain. So, in addition to these lower back exercises, it is also important to perform the alignment exercises (pp. 43–45) on a daily basis.

———— **PRECAUTION** ————

In order to avoid pressure on the lower back and chronic lower back pain, the following exercises should be avoided:

The straight-leg, flat-back position
The double leg lift
The straight-leg sit-up
The straight-leg toe touch
The yoga plow
The windmill
The unsupported lateral stretch

Exercises to Avoid

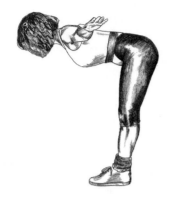

Straight leg, flat back

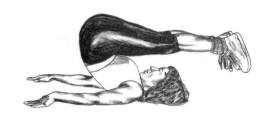

Yoga plow

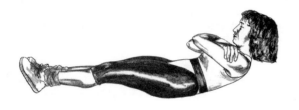

Straight-leg sit-up

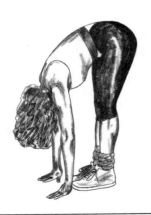

Straight-leg toe touch

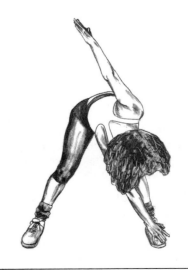

Windmill

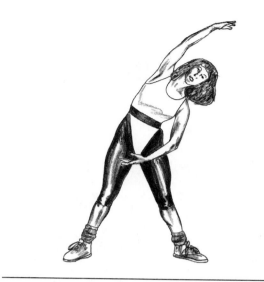

Unsupported lateral stretch

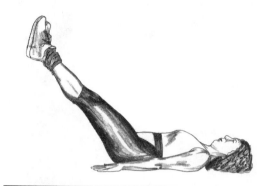

Double leg lift

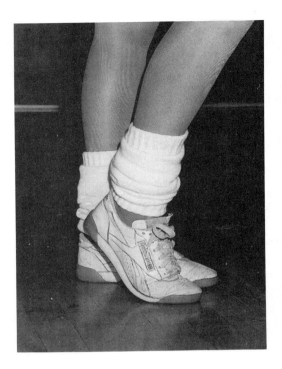
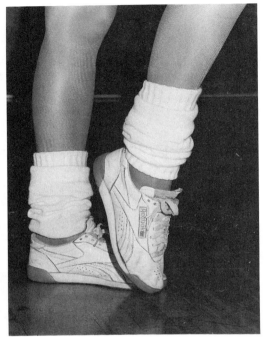
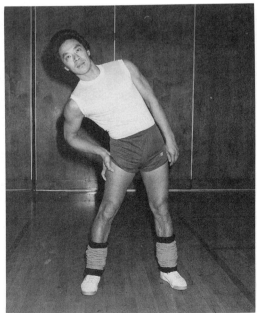
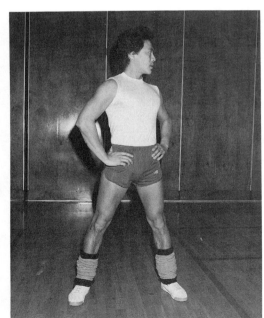

Warm-up

Chapter

7

A warm-up is like tuning a fine instrument. The body, the aerobics dancer's instrument, must be tuned in preparation to responding to the demands placed on it in an aerobic dance workout.

Most professionals highly recommend the warm-up, although there is little scientific evidence that it helps performance or prevents injury. However, the warm-up is stressed for several reasons. First, it is believed that warm-up shortens the cardiovascular and muscular systems' adjustment period to the oncoming stress of physical activity. The warm-up thus lets the body gradually shift from a resting state to an active state without undue shock.

Second, the warm-up is thought to minimize the risk of inadequate blood flow to the heart during the first few seconds of heavy exercise because it gives the heart time to adjust from being at rest to undergoing sudden, strenuous activity (7). This also helps to prevent arrhythmia (abnormal heartbeats) because the blood supply has time to change to the greater demand placed on it.

The third major goal of the warm-up is to raise the body's core temperature by as much as 2 degrees. This can affect the body in many ways:

1. Increases the metabolic rate, which in turn increases the rate at which energy is used
2. Increases the flow of blood to the muscles
3. Increases the release of oxygen to the muscles
4. Increases the speed and force of muscle contraction
5. Increases muscle elasticity

Finally, the warm-up is also thought to be of important psychological benefit because it mentally prepares a person for the strenuous demands of the upcoming workout. Many experts believe that exercise prior to a strenuous activity gradually prepares a person to go all out without fear of injury. In competitive athletics, many participants consider the warm-up an activity that prepares them mentally for their event, an opportunity for them to clearly focus their concentration or to psyche up for the upcoming performance (38).

WARM-UP CONCEPTS

We believe that a warm-up is valuable before engaging in a vigorous aerobic dance workout. To attain a thorough warm-up, you should adhere to certain concepts. The warm-up is *not* a time for intense stretching; it is a time to loosen and ready the muscles for the aerobic dances to follow.

The warm-up consists of three phases:

1. Isolations
2. Active warm-up
3. Static stretch

The first phase is very short and involves simple isolation moves and concentrates on posture and body alignment. This phase may take no more than 1 to 2 minutes and is basically used as an introduction for movement.

The second phase is termed the active warm-up and involves simple calisthenics, full-body movements, and possibly light jogging or walking movements around the classroom. During the active warm-up, start slowly and gradually increase the pace and intensity of the movements until your body begins to feel loose and warm. Low-impact movements such as marching, light jogging, knee lifts, grapevines, the charleston, schottische, and jazz square are appropriate for the active warm-up (see Chapter 8 for a complete description of these movements). The active warm-up elevates your heart rate and warms the muscles. Light perspiration may be an indicator that your muscles are ready for the next phase.

The final phase of the warm-up is called the static stretch. A **static stretch** is when you extend a specific part of the body to the point of slight discomfort and hold this position for 10 to 30 seconds. Exercise stretches should be static rather than **ballistic** (bouncing). A slow static stretch tends to counteract a muscle's stretch reflex, whereas the sudden stretch of a ballistic exercise contracts the muscle, which negates the purpose of the stretch (22). In addition, static stretching requires less expenditure of energy, which probably causes less muscle soreness and yields more relief from muscular distress (18).

The static stretch phase consists of simple stretches of specific muscle groups used in aerobic dance. These muscle groups include the quadriceps (front of the thigh), the hamstrings (back of the thigh), the calf muscles (back of the lower leg), the shins (front of the lower leg), the shoulders, and the lower back.

The time necessary for warm-up varies with each individual, depending on fitness level and age. Generally, a minimum warm-up of 5 to 10 minutes is adequate. Pre-warm-up exercises can help those who want more warm-up activity. For such individual pre-warm-up, allow yourself approximately 10 minutes before class. Use the simple exercises described in this chapter, and be sure to pay extra attention to warming up any area of your body that is weak or prone to injury.

ISOLATION EXERCISES

Neck

NECK ISOLATIONS

Drop your chin down. Tilt your head from side to side. Look to your right and left.

———————— **PRECAUTION** ————————

Head circles (not included in this text) have been identified as a contraindicated exercise; they can put undue stress on the cervical spine and should be avoided.

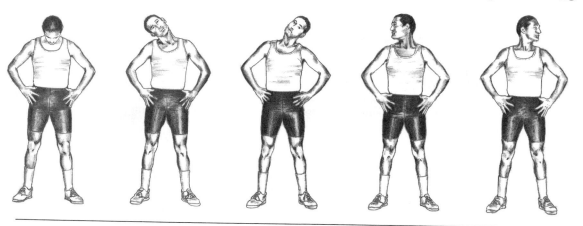

Neck isolations

Shoulders

SHOULDER SHRUGS

Elevate your shoulders to your ears and then press your shoulders down. Lift both shoulders together and then one shoulder at a time.

SHOULDER CIRCLES

Because most people have a slight case of round shoulders due to desk work, housework, or other occupational situations, forward shoulder circles are not a necessary isolation exercise. Rather, to alleviate this problem, the isolation movement is performed in the backward direction. Be sure to go through the entire range of motion and use this exercise to relax the shoulder region.

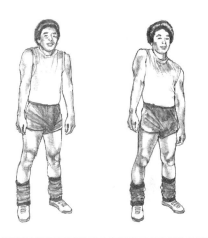

Shoulder shrugs

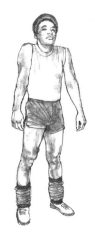

Shoulder circles

Rib Cage

RIB ISOLATIONS

Place your hands on your shoulders to isolate the movement to your ribs and no other parts of the body. Move your ribs to the right, left, forward, and backward. This movement can be performed in place or with small steps in any direction.

Hips

HIP ISOLATIONS

Bend your knees, with your hands in any position. Move your hips left, right, forward, and backward. You can also move your hips in a circular direction and with the feet traveling in any direction.

ACTIVE WARM-UP MOVEMENTS

The movements and steps used in the active warm-up are described and illustrated in the next chapter. The main idea for this phase of the warm-up is to begin moving around the classroom with moderate, level movements. The vocabulary of movements for aerobic dance continues to grow, and each aerobics instructor will present specific movements for this phase of the warm-up that suit his or her individual style.

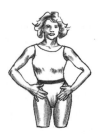 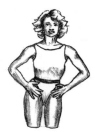 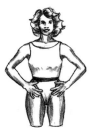 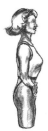 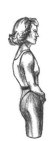

Rib isolations

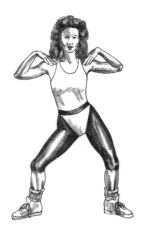 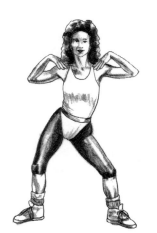 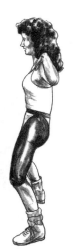 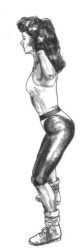

Hip isolations

STATIC STRETCHES

Shoulders and Chest

CHEST STRETCH

Clasp your hands behind your back and stretch your chest muscles by pulling your shoulder blades together. You can also perform the chest stretch while bending forward at your waist and lifting your clasped hands away from your lower back, toward the ceiling.

ACROSS-THE-BODY STRETCH

In a standing position, with your feet shoulder width apart, or sitting cross-legged on the floor, keep your spine erect as you cross your right arm in front of your body and take hold of it with your left hand. Gently stretch your arm as close to your body as possible. Do not elevate your arm above your chest. You can perform this same stretch with your left arm over your head and your right arm gently stretching it by holding it at the upper arm or by the hand. Both versions of this stretch should be felt at the back of your arm and the upper parts of your shoulder and back. Repeat the stretch on your other side.

Upper Back

UPPER BACK STRETCHES

In a standing position, with your feet shoulder width apart and your knees slightly bent, clasp your hands in front of your body and press your palms forward. For another upper back stretch, maintain the same standing position and wrap

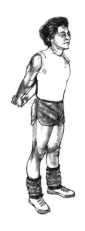

Chest stretch

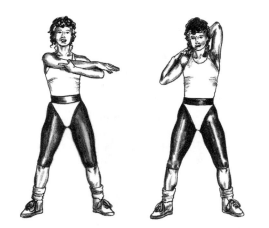

Across-the-body stretch

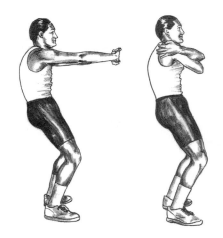

Upper back stretches

your arms around your body as if you were giving yourself a hug.

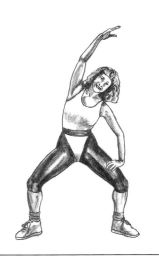

Lateral stretch

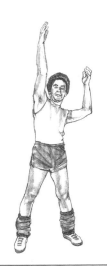

Reach stretch

———— **MOVEMENT TIPS** ————

- Keep the pelvis tucked under in this position so you can also feel the stretch at the lower back.
- Keep your abdominals tight while holding this stretch.

Rib Cage and Waist

LATERAL STRETCH

Stand with your feet shoulder width apart. Raise one arm over your head and bend *sideways* from your waist. Be sure you do not lean forward or backward; bend directly sideways. Do not move below your waist. To protect your lower back, support your trunk with your other hand on your thigh or your forearm on your thigh, keeping your knees slightly bent. You can perform this exercise with a variety of arm positions and from a sitting position.

———— **PRECAUTIONS** ————

- Be sure to bend your knees slightly when performing this exercise.
- Contract your abdominals so that there is minimal stress on the lower back.
- Always support the stretch by placing one hand on your thigh.

REACH STRETCH

Reach up to the ceiling with one arm at a time. Fully stretch your side and rib cage. Do not hyperextend your rib cage or your lower back.

———— **PRECAUTION** ————

Since the aim of the reach stretch is to stretch the sides of the body, try not to elevate or tense the shoulders.

Hips and Buttocks

WIDE AND DEEP KNEE BEND

Stand in a wide straddle position, with your legs turned out from your hip joints. Bend deeply at your knees, keeping your heels flat on the ground. Press your thighs open with your elbows.

—— PRECAUTIONS ——

- In this position, be sure to keep your knees in line with your toes to avoid stress on the knee ligaments.
- To protect the knees from strain, avoid dropping your pelvis below knee level.

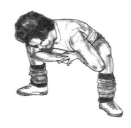

Wide and deep knee bend

LOOSE SWING

Stand with your feet together and parallel. Stretch your arms toward the ceiling and then swing your arms forward and down, releasing your upper body while bending your knees. Return to the starting position by swinging your arms and body upward and straightening your legs. Perform the exercise slowly.

—— PRECAUTIONS ——

- Attempt to keep your knees in line with your toes rather than letting the knees come together.
- Allow your body to relax, but keep your abdominal muscles contracted.

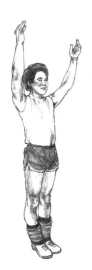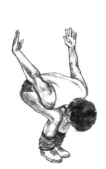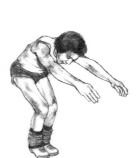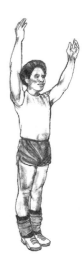

Loose swing

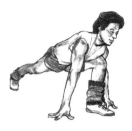

Runner lunge

Upper Legs

RUNNER LUNGE

From a deep lunge position, with your feet parallel, place your hands on the floor on either side of or on the inside of your forward, bent knee. In this position, the heel of your front foot must remain on the floor; your back leg should be straight with your foot fully flexed and your toes pressed against the floor.

——————— **PRECAUTION** ———————

Be sure your knee is directly over your ankle in this position. If your knee extends over or beyond your toes, there will be unnecessary stress on the knee ligament.

SIDE LUNGE

Stand in a wide straddle position with your legs turned out from your hip joints and your hands on your thighs. Lunge by bending one knee and keeping your other leg straight. You can lift the heel of your bent leg or keep it on the floor. If you lift your heel, the stretch will be emphasized on the inner thigh of your straight leg. If you keep the heel on the floor, the stretch will also involve the calf muscles of your bent leg. Make sure you do not compress your knee more than 90 degrees. You can also perform this exercise with your hands on the floor for balance. You can use your arms to help keep your bent knee directly over your ankle.

——————— **PRECAUTIONS** ———————

- As in the runner lunge position, keep your bent knee in line with your ankle.
- Your body weight should be between the two legs; think of keeping the pelvis between the heels as opposed to "sitting" on the heel of the lunged knee.

QUADRICEP STRETCH

You can perform this exercise in a variety of positions. The main idea is to bend your lower leg

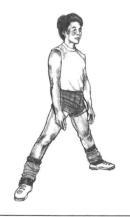
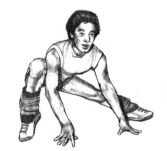
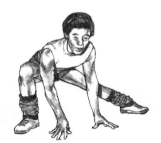

Side lunge

behind your body with the sole of your foot reaching toward the ceiling. Hold the lifted foot with your hand and stretch it toward your buttocks (refer to the *Quadricep stretch* illustration and *movement tips* below for additional positions).

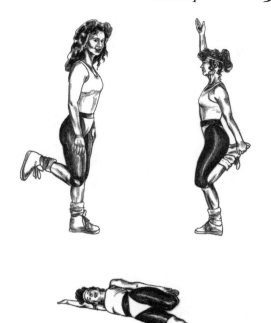

MOVEMENT TIPS

- You can do this exercise on the floor, lying either on your stomach with your leg pulled back or on your side with the top leg being stretched.
- For the less flexible individual, stand with your back to the wall. Place one foot against the wall, keeping your bent leg at a 90-degree angle.
- You can also perform this exercise with a partner, placing your free hand on the other person's shoulder for balance.

PRECAUTION

- If you feel pain in your bent knee, discontinue this exercise.
- Maintain proper alignment when performing this exercise.

Quadricep stretch

HAMSTRING STRETCH

Stand with your feet shoulder width apart and extend one foot in front of the other in a parallel position. Bend your supporting leg and keep your front leg straight, with the foot flexed. Place both hands on your thighs for upper body support.

MOVEMENT TIP

Flex your foot as much as possible to achieve the maximum stretch.

PRECAUTIONS

- Tighten your abdominals to relieve lower back strain.
- Do not hyperextend the straight leg.
- Keep your weight centered between your feet.

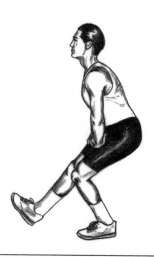

Hamstring stretch

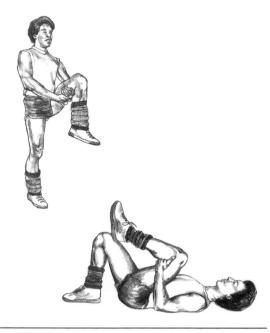

Knee lift stretch

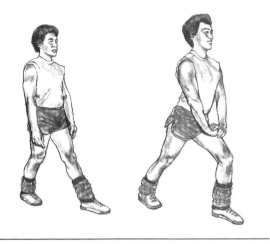

Calf stretch

KNEE LIFT STRETCH

Stand with your feet parallel and pull one knee to your chest, holding your leg underneath the thigh. You can also perform this stretch while lying on the floor with bent legs together. Pull one knee to your chest, holding your leg under the knee. This exercise stretches the hamstrings, gluteals, and lower back muscles.

———— PRECAUTIONS ————

- In both positions, be sure to relax your supporting leg to alleviate any stress on the lower back.
- In both positions, attempt to maintain correct alignment.
- In the lying position, do not grasp the knee as it may cause undue stress on the knee joint.

Lower Legs

CALF STRETCH

Stand with your feet together and parallel. Step with one foot forward so that your feet are approximately 1 to 2 feet apart. Lunge onto your front leg, being sure to keep your back leg straight and your back toes directed forward. Keep both heels on the floor. You can rest your hands on your front leg as an added weight to stretch your back leg.

———— PRECAUTIONS ————

- The back heel must remain in contact with the floor in order to achieve the maximum stretch.
- Keep your bent knee in line with your ankle.

SOLEUS STRETCH

Maintain the same standing position used for the calf stretch but bend your back knee. Your back foot may be positioned closer to your front foot if necessary. Your back heel must remain on the ground. Your hands can be placed in any of the fundamental stretching positions.

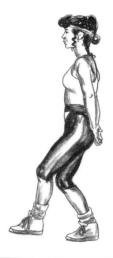

Soleus stretch

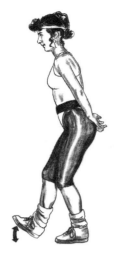

Toe tap

TOE TAP

You can perform this exercise in many positions. In one common position, stand with your feet about 1 foot apart and your legs turned out from the hip joints. Tap your forward foot about 8 to 10 times and then repeat on the other side. You can also turn your foot out and in on alternating toe taps. This exercise warms up the shin muscle, tibialis anterior. The toe tap can also be performed in the runner lunge position as an added warm-up to the hip flexors.

Ankles

ANKLE FLEXION AND EXTENSION

Standing or sitting, flex (point your foot up) and then extend (point your foot down) your ankle slowly.

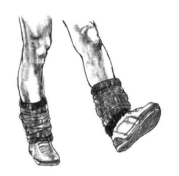

Ankle flexion

——————— PRECAUTION ———————

When flexing or extending your ankles, maintain a straight line from your big toe to your ankle to avoid toeing in and excessively stretching the muscles on the outside of your ankle.

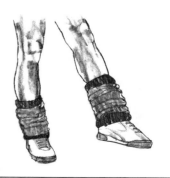

Ankle extension

ANKLE CIRCLE

Standing or sitting, slowly circle your ankle with your foot flexed and then with your foot extended.

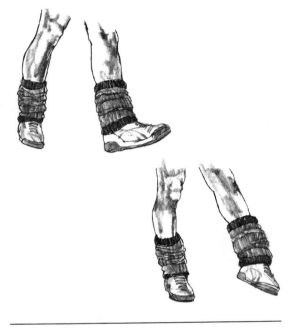

Ankle circle

WARM-UP ROUTINES AND PRECAUTIONS

The exercises described can be combined in many ways. For maximum benefit, you must perform repetitions of each exercise. When you are creating routines, it is important that transitions between exercises be smooth and flow naturally. Music for warm-up routines can be any Top 40 favorite, as long as it has a steady, rhythmic beat and preferably a 4/4 time signature or one that can be counted in 4 or 8 beats. The beats per minute should be between 120 and 140.

Warm-up exercises should begin slowly. Gradually increase your effort until you reach moderate pace and intensity. Choose rhythmic movements that flow from one sequence to the next. Keep your hips stable when performing exercises involving a lateral stretch or twisting of the torso. Always include exercises for the Achilles tendons, calf muscles, lower back, quadriceps, hamstrings, and shoulder joints since these body parts are heavily used in aerobic dance. The warm-up should last 5 to 10 minutes. Immediately begin your aerobic workout when you complete your warm-up routine so that you do not lose the benefits of the warm-up. Finally and most importantly, remember that the warm-up must do just that—warm you up and prepare you for the vigorous workout ahead!

The following routines work with any song that can be counted in 4 or 8 beats. The musical choice is your own; just be sure it is upbeat yet not too fast and is something that inspires you to move!

WARM-UP ROUTINE

Movement	Repetitions	Counts
ISOLATIONS		
Neck isolations	8	4 each
Shoulder shrugs	8	4 each
Shoulder circles (backward)	4	4 each
Reach stretch	8, alternating right and left	2 each
ACTIVE WARM-UP		
March in place	8	1 each
3 walks and a hop (schottische; see Chapter 8)	1 time forward and backward	4 each
Grapevine and a clap (see Chapter 8)	4, alternating right and left	4 each
Jazz square (see Chapter 8)	2	4 each
Repeat from "March in place"	3 sets	
STATIC STRETCHES		
Lateral stretch	2, alternating right and left	8 each
Across-the-body stretch	Alternate right and left	8 each
Chest stretch	2	8 each
Calf stretch	1 right	16
Soleus stretch	1 right	16
Hamstring stretch	1 right	16
Runner lunge	1 right	16
Quadricep stretch	1 right	16
Repeat on left side from "Calf stretch"		
Toe tap with feet in wide position	8 right, 8 left	1 each

March it out and begin aerobics!

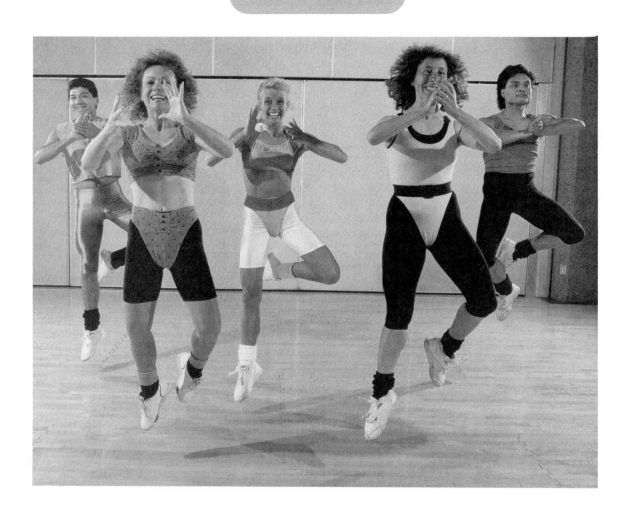

Aerobic Dances

Chapter

Aerobic dances consist of steps and movements drawn from pedestrian locomotor movements that are performed to music and are stylized after a variety of dance forms, including jazz, ballet, modern, folk, square, and social dance. Aerobic dance movements, done during the aerobic session of the class, must be performed *nonstop* for a minimum of 15 minutes and must sustain an individual's target heart rate. You must pace yourself so that you can complete the entire aerobic section of the workout. If you find yourself tiring, slow down, but *never* come to a complete stop. *Reminder:* Carefully monitor your target heart rate by taking your pulse after the first dance and then periodically throughout the rest of the session.

This chapter describes locomotor movements and dance steps commonly used in aerobic dances, discusses combinations of these move-ments, and outlines precautions to follow in the aerobic dance class. A discussion of how to choreograph an aerobic dance routine and several examples of such routines are also included.

LOCOMOTOR MOVEMENTS

The basic locomotor movements used in aerobic dance are walking, running, jumping, hopping, leaping, skipping, and sliding. Variations of these move-ments are created by integrating arm and footwork patterns and directional changes; the variations are then enlivened with snaps, claps, and body slaps.

Walking

A walk is a transfer of weight from one foot to the other, with one foot always on the ground.

Variations

Walking in place
Walking forward
Walking backward
Walking diagonally
Walking in a circle
Turning
Walking on your toes
Walking forward, stepping together; walking backward, stepping together; walking sideways, stepping together
Walking in a square

Grapevine:
1. Step to the left with your left foot.
2. Step to the left with your right foot crossing in front of your left foot.
3. Step to the left with your left foot.
4. Step to the left with your right foot crossing behind your left foot.

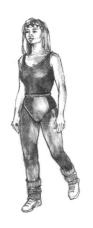
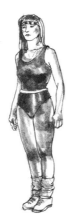

Walking forward, stepping together

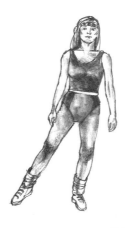

Walking sideways, right foot to side

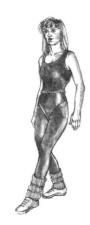
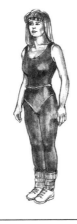

Walking backward, stepping together

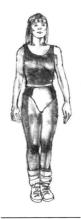
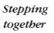
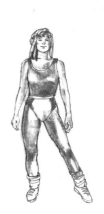

Stepping together

Walking sideways, left foot to side

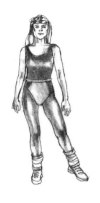 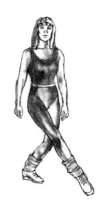 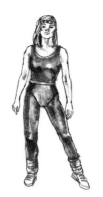 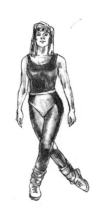

Grapevine

Running

A run is a transfer of weight from one foot to the other. At one point in a run, both feet are off the ground. A run is faster than a walk.

Variations

Running in place
Running forward
Running backward
Running diagonally
Running in a circle
Running in a figure eight
High-knee runs

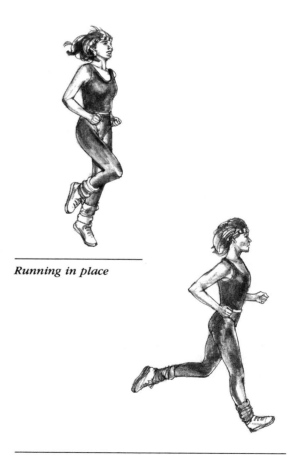

Running in place

Running forward

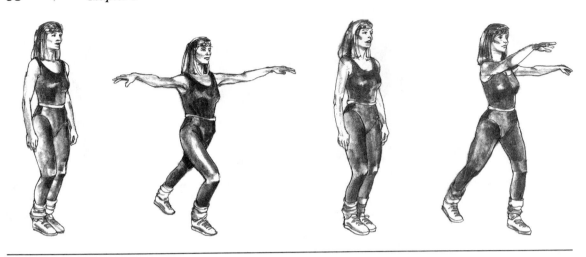

Scissors jumping jacks

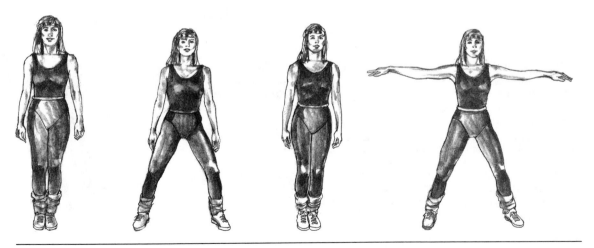

Progressive jumping jacks

Jumping

A jump is an aerial movement in which a person takes off from two feet and lands on two feet.

Variations

Jumping in place
Jumping forward
Jumping backward
Jumping sideways
Jumping diagonally
Quarter, half, and whole turns
Regular jumping jacks
Scissors jumping jacks:

1. Jump with your feet together.
2. Jump with your legs splitting front and back; swing your arms in opposition.
3. Jump with your feet together; bring your arms to your sides.
4. Alternate legs on the split jump.

Crossover jumping jacks:

1. Jump to a straddle position.
2. Jump crossing your legs.
3. Alternate crossing your legs first in front and then in back.

Progressive jumping jacks:

1. Jump with your feet together.
2. Jump to a straddle position.
3. Jump with your feet together.
4. Jump to a straddle position; raise your arms to shoulder height.
5. Jump with your feet together; bring your arms down to your sides.
6. Jump to a straddle position; clap your hands overhead.
7. Jump with your feet together; bring your arms down to your sides.
8. Perform the above sequence in reverse order.

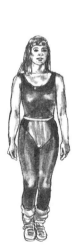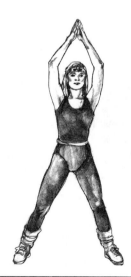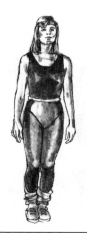

Progressive jumping jacks (continued)

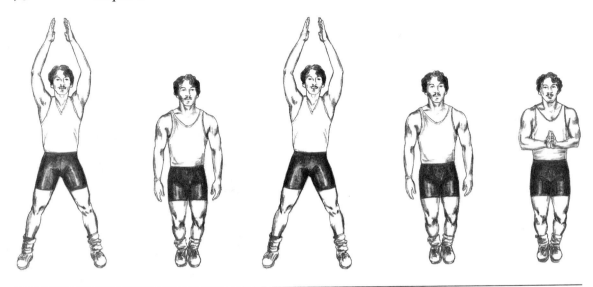

Rhythm jacks

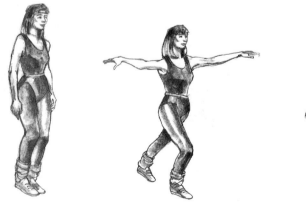

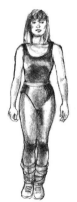

Jump lunge forward or backward

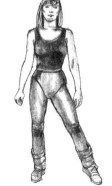

Jump lunge sideways

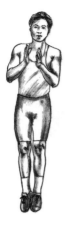 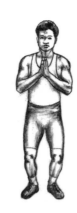 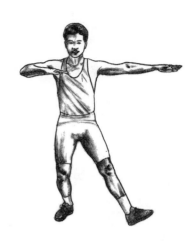

Breakaway

Rhythm jacks:
1. Jump to a straddle position; clap your hands overhead.
2. Jump with your feet together; bring your arms down to your sides.
3. Jump to a straddle position; clap your hands overhead.
4. Jump with your feet together; bring your arms down to your sides.
5. Jump in place with your feet together 4 times, clapping on each jump.

Jump lunge: Alternately jump in place and then jump to a lunge position forward, backward, or sideways.

Breakaway:
1. Jump with your feet together; clap your hands.
2. Jump, extending one leg to the side, touching the heel of your extended leg to the floor; push your arm on the same side as the extended leg straight out to the side, and bend your other arm at the elbow at shoulder height.
3. Jump, your feet together, and repeat the exercise on your other side.

—————— **MOVEMENT TIP** ——————

In rhythm jacks, you can either clap your hands overhead or raise your arms to shoulder height. Choreographed arm movements may be added for diversity.

—————— **PRECAUTION** ——————

Always land from a jump with your knees bent. Land on the balls of your feet and press your heels down to make complete contact with the floor to absorb the shock of the jump, to avoid placing stress on the knees, and to stretch the Achilles tendons.

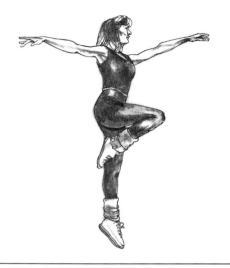

Hopping

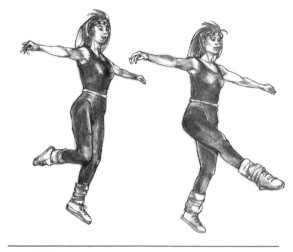

Hop-kick

Hopping

A hop is an aerial movement in which a person takes off on one foot and lands on that same foot.

Variations

Hopping in place
Hopping forward
Hopping backward

Hopping diagonally

Hop-kick: Bend your lifted leg in and then kick to the front or side.

Can-can:

1. Circle your lifted leg from your knee in front of your body.
2. Bend your lifted leg sideways and circle from your knee.

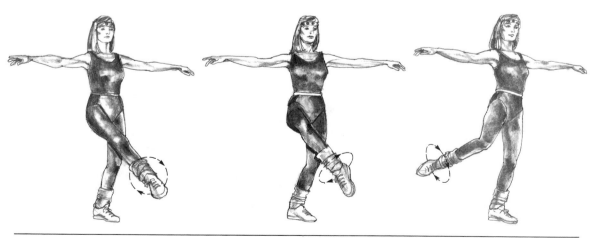

Can-can

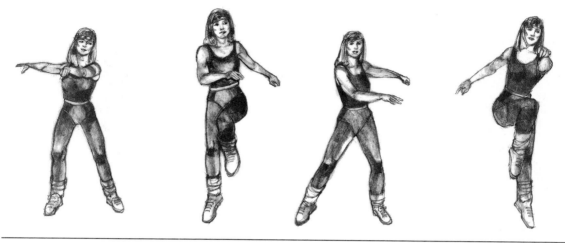

Flea-hop

3. Lift your bent leg behind your body and circle from your knee.

Flea-hop:
1. Hop on one leg, lifting the opposite knee to hip height; swing arms in opposition.
2. Repeat this hop, alternating legs.

Pendulum hop:
1. Hop on one leg, extending your other leg to the side at a 45-degree angle.
2. Repeat this hop, alternating legs.

———— **M O V E M E N T   T I P** ————

Pendulum hops may be performed as double hops or single hops or a combination of both.

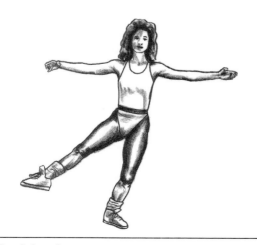
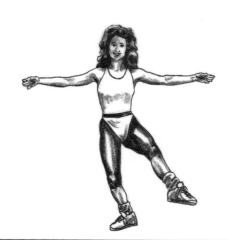

Pendulum hop

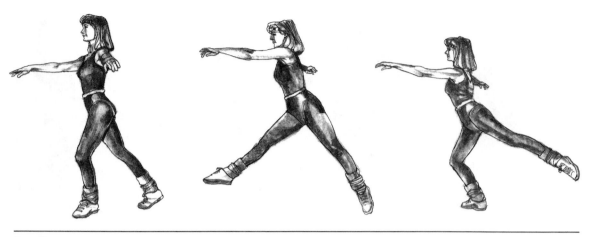

Leaping

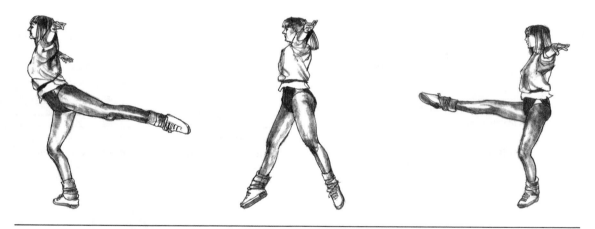

Leaping backward

Leaping

A leap is an aerial movement in which a person moves from one foot to the other. Between the takeoff and landing, the body is suspended in air.

Variations

Leaping forward
Leaping backward
Leaping sideways
Leaping diagonally
Rocking:
1. Leap forward onto one leg.
2. Immediately leap backward onto your opposite leg. (You can also rock from side to side.)

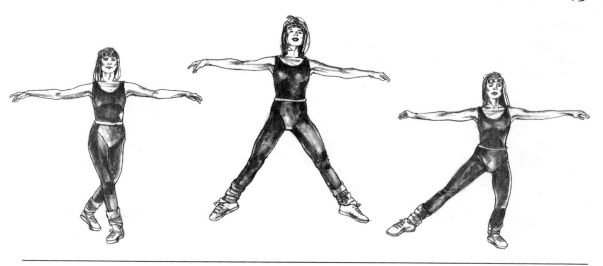

Leaping sideways

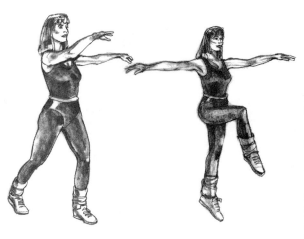

Skipping

Skipping

A skip is a combination of a step and a hop on the same foot, with an uneven rhythmic pattern.

Variations

Skipping forward
Skipping backward
Skipping sideways
Skipping in a circle
Turning

Sliding

A slide, or chassé, is a smooth, gliding, step-together step. At its peak, the body is suspended in the air, with the legs together and fully extended.

Variations

Sliding forward
Sliding backward
Sliding sideways

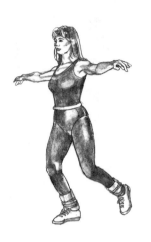
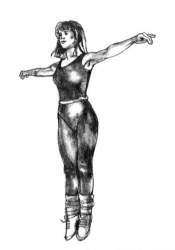
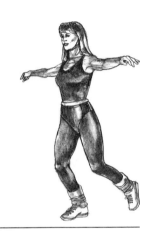

Sliding

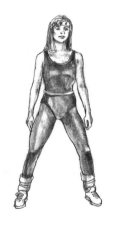
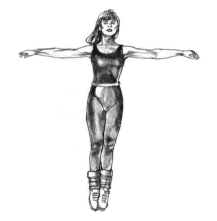
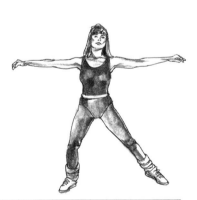

Sliding sideways

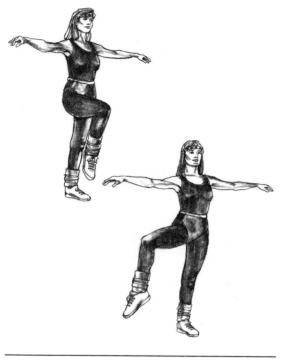

Knee lifts

DANCE STEPS

The following movements originate from various dance forms. This brief selection is not inclusive; it is representative of the endless number of dance steps available for aerobic routines.

Jazz and Modern Dance

KNEE LIFTS

Perform to the front or to the side.

KICKS

Perform to the front, back, or side.

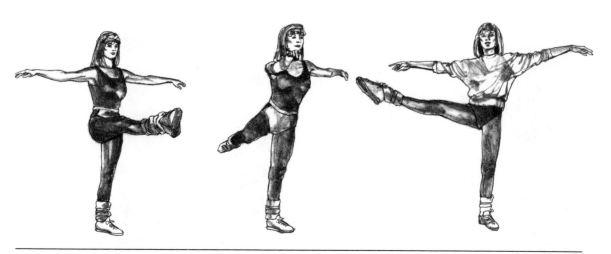

Kicks

KICK BALL CHANGE

Kick one leg to the front; then step to the rear of your supporting leg, placing your weight on the ball of your foot, with your heel lifted. Your other foot then steps in place, with your weight transfering onto this foot.

JAZZ SQUARE

The jazz square consists of four walking steps performed in a square pattern. Step forward with your right foot. Cross your left foot in front of your right. Step back on your right foot. Step to the left with your left foot. This step can start on either foot.

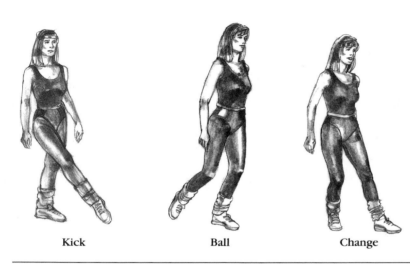

Kick   Ball   Change

Kick ball change

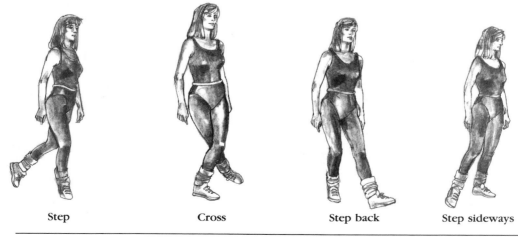

Step   Cross   Step back   Step sideways

Jazz square

PIVOT

Perform the pivot on two feet, quickly shifting your body to face in the opposite direction. Both of your feet remain on the floor in their positions as you pivot your body.

PADDLE TURN

The paddle turn is a simple turn that pivots your body around on one spot. Your weight shifts from one foot to the other. Your supporting, stationary leg pivots on the ball of the foot, with your heel lifting slightly off the floor. Your other leg extends to the side and "paddles" on the ball of the foot, rotating your body in a circular direction while your foot traces an imaginary circular pattern on the floor.

MOVEMENT TIP

To get exact quarter turns, imagine a clock on the floor. Your "paddle" foot must touch at twelve o'clock, three o'clock, six o'clock, and nine o'clock.

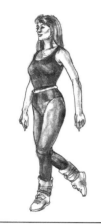
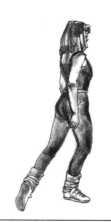

Pivot

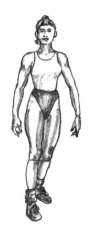
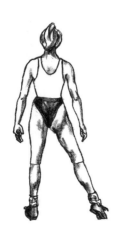
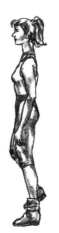
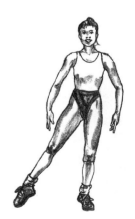

Paddle turn

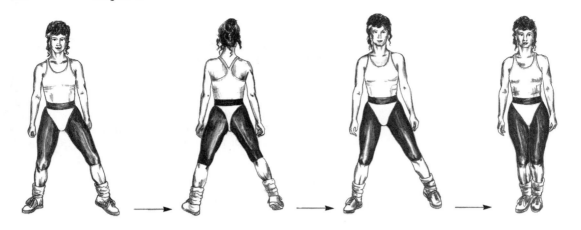

Three-step turn

THREE-STEP TURN

Begin by stepping to the side. Step and rotate 180 degrees to face the back. Step and rotate 180 degrees to face the front. End the turn by bringing your feet together or touching the final stepping foot to the other foot.

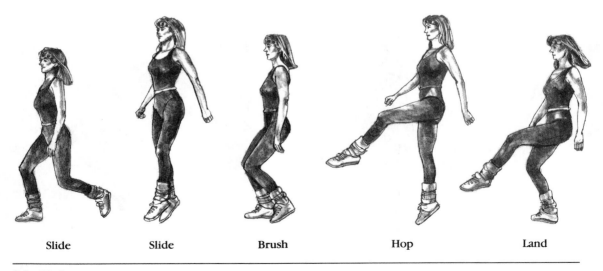

| Slide | Slide | Brush | Hop | Land |

Schottische

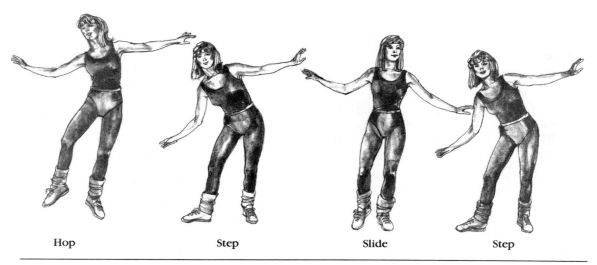

Hop   Step   Slide   Step

Polka

Folk Dance

SCHOTTISCHE

A schottische is a forward slide, or chassé, combined with a brush-hop. Brush your back foot forward, slightly off the floor, on the hop. Make your hop on the same foot as the one you used for the step.

POLKA

A polka is a hop on one foot, with a quick, bouncy side slide, or chassé. The polka can also be done from side to side and while turning.

HEEL-TOE POLKA

Hop on your left foot, and place your right heel on the floor in front of your body. Cross your right foot behind your left foot, placing your right toe on the floor. Continue the polka step with the side slide described above.

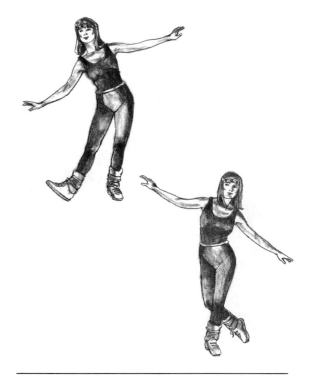

Heel-toe polka

SQUARE DANCE

Square dance movements are performed with a partner.

DO-SI-DO

Face your partner and run around each other in a circle without turning your bodies. Midway through your circle, you and your partner will be back to back.

SWING YOUR PARTNER

Link right elbows with your partner and swing for 8 to 16 counts. Then link your left elbows and swing in the opposite direction.

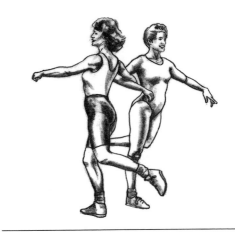

Swing your partner

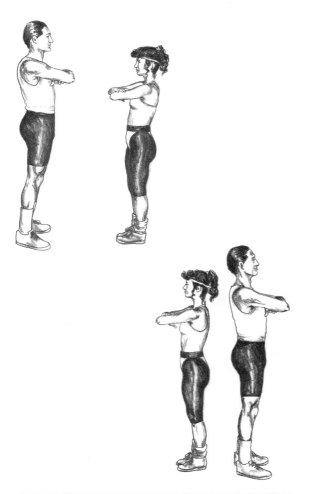

Do-si-do

Social Dance

CHA-CHA

The cha-cha is a combination of 2 slow steps, 2 quick steps, and a final slow step. The rhythm is 1-2-3 and 4. Step forward onto the full foot with your knees bent. Step back onto the ball of your opposite foot. On the triple "cha-cha-cha" steps, keep your knees bent and sway your hips, stepping in place or traveling very little. In aerobic dance, the cha-cha is modified with large step movements and traveling patterns (forward, backward, or sideways) to increase intensity.

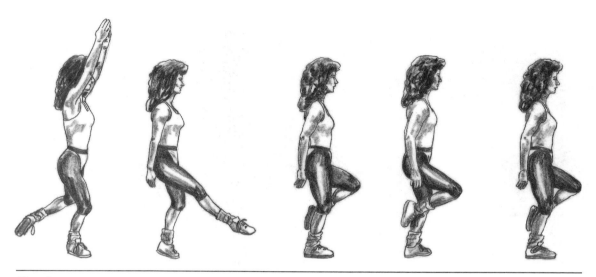

Cha-cha

CHARLESTON

Step forward onto your right foot. Swing your left leg forward to touch the floor with the ball of your left foot ahead of your right foot. Step backward with your left foot. Swing your right leg back to touch the floor with the ball of your right foot behind your left foot. You may kick your leg instead of touching your foot to the floor to increase the intensity of the movement.

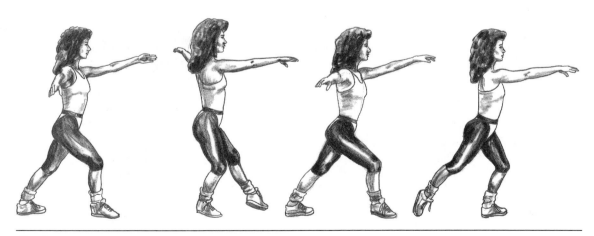

Charleston

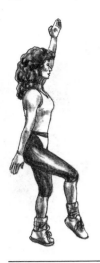 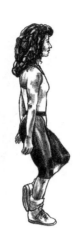 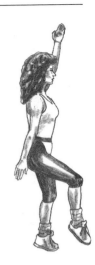

Pony

PONY

The pony is a combination of a small sideways leap and a ball change. Leap sideways right onto your right foot. Step onto the ball of your left foot. Quickly shift your body weight by stepping onto your right foot (change). Reverse the pony by leaping from your right foot to your left foot. The pony is done with bouncy stepping movements to increase intensity and a variety of foot patterns with the pull-change to add interest and variety.

ARM MOVEMENTS

You can perform variations of the basic movements by applying arm patterns. Those commonly used in aerobic dance include:

Arm circles—make small or large circles with your arms extended to the side and at shoulder height.

Arm scissors—alternately cross your straight arms in front or in back of your body.

Arm reaches—reach up, to the side, or down or do a combination of all three movements.

Karate punches—punch each of your arms diagonally across your body.

Pectoral press—hold your arms out to the side and bent upward from your elbows. Bring your forearms together in front of your face, elbows and wrists touching. Open your arms to the starting position.

Coordination arms—stretch your arms straight out in front of your chest. Open your arms out to the side. Close your arms at chest height. Drop your arms straight down to slap the top of your thighs. This is a 4-count movement.

Latin Roll—keeping your arms bent at the elbows, roll your forearms in a circular fashion around one another. Vary the roll at chest level, waist level, and above the head.

Pat-a-cake—clap your hands together close to your chest. Push your right arm forward horizontally at chest height. Clap. Push your left arm forward horizontally at chest height. Clap. Push both arms forward horizontally at chest height. Clap. Clap. (Clap twice.)

PRECAUTION —————

Avoid arm movements that violently fling your arms beyond the line of your shoulders, causing the chest muscles to overstretch.

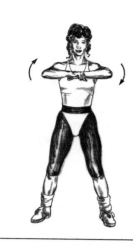

Latin roll

COMBINATIONS OF MOVEMENTS

Just as the locomotor and dance step movements are endless, so too are the combinations of these movements. Listed are a few simple combinations derived from the steps already described. All of these can be adapted to an intensity appropriate to your fitness level. Kicks can be performed high or low; running can be geared to a low-impact level; and knee lifts can be done without jumping.

3 walks or runs and a hop accented with a snap.

3 walks or runs and a jump accented with a clap.

3 walks or runs with a kick, with arms reaching either vertically or horizontally.

3 walks or runs and a pivot.

Jump reach—jump followed by a hop with your leg extending to the side and your arms reaching diagonally away from your extended leg.

Hopscotch—a combination of a jump and a hop, with your lifted leg crossing behind your hopping leg. This movement alternates hopping feet.

Jump-kick—your kicking leg can kick to the front, side, or back. You can use a variety of arm patterns or perform claps under or over your leg.

Knee lift then jump-kick-jump.

Hop, touching your heel with your opposite hand, then jump-hop combined with a knee lift-jump.

PRECAUTIONS, OR HOW TO SURVIVE THE AEROBIC DANCE CLASS!

Before we describe aerobic dance routines, you should be aware of how to get the most out of your class and avoid complications. Always monitor your heart rate to make sure you are working at your target heart rate. If you have mastered taking your pulse easily, you should continue to walk while monitoring your heart rate. Begin your aerobic workout section at a low intensity; gradually increase and sustain the intensity as you reach your target heart rate. Make sure you are breathing evenly throughout the dances. *Do not hold your breath!*

You should be able to talk while performing the dances. If you are unable to carry on a conversation, you are working too hard. Make sure you *land with your knees bent* on all jumps, hops, leaps, and other aerial movements. Do *not* land with straight legs. Do not perform jogs and runs flat-footed. Your landing must be cushioned by rolling through your foot. Never come to a complete stop during the aerobic section of class except in the event of injury. Slow down to a walking pace if you are out of breath.

Slow down immediately if you feel a side stitch or leg cramps. If the cramp does not stop after you slow the pace, stop and stretch and/or massage the area in pain. If you injure yourself during the dances, seek first aid attention immediately. *Stop* if you feel chest pain, irregular heart rate rhythm, dizziness, or nausea.

Aerobic dance is a time to strive toward your physical fitness goals; it is also a time to have fun. Overload, but do not overdo. Remember, this is not a competition; success means to *keep moving!*

AEROBIC DANCE ROUTINES

Aerobic dance routines are the main challenge and excitement of the aerobic dance class because they enable participants to "dance their hearts out." Aerobic dance routines are performed to popular songs that have a steady beat and lively tempo. The steps and movements are usually counted and choreographed in beats of 8: for example, jog 8 counts, jump 8 counts, hop and kick 8 counts, and so on.

A *phrase* of aerobic dance movements is a combination of two or more sets of 8 counts; thus you have 16, 24, 32, and so on counts of music. The choreography of an aerobic dance consists of several movement phrases repeated many times throughout the dance. A change in phrase in an aerobic dance routine is often determined by the music. For example, a phrase is performed and repeated every time the chorus of a song is repeated. A different phrase is used for the verse, instrumental, and/or introductory part of the music. This division of music gives continuity to the dance and makes it easy for the dancers to remember and follow.

Most aerobic dance routines are performed with the leader at the front of the class and the group facing the leader, but variations of group formations add novelty to the daily workout regimens. Dances can be performed in a circle, with a partner, or in two lines facing each other (such as the Virginia reel). Group interaction can add much energy to the class and encourage a sense of classroom community. The instructor should not always be performing with the class; in addition to leading aerobic dance routines, it is the instructor's responsibility to correct posture and alignment, to assist students with the execution of steps, and to monitor, as much as possible, individual pace.

CHOREOGRAPHING AN AEROBIC DANCE ROUTINE

The aerobic dance routine must be vigorous enough to sustain your pulse at its target range. Although this is the most important requirement of an aerobic dance routine, the routine should also be fun to perform, with a variety of easy-to-remember movements and dance steps. After all, during the aerobic dance routine, your main goal is to *keep moving!*

Choreographing an aerobic dance routine follows certain logical steps: selecting the music, analyzing the music, and developing dance movements suitable to the music. The same choreographic principles can be used for all phases of aerobic dance, that is, warm-up, low-impact, peak aerobic, and cool-down aerobic routines.

Music Selection

The selection of music is the first decision. It is vital that the music inspire movement because it is the basic motivation for an aerobic dance. The music should be upbeat with a steady tempo.

Each phase of the aerobic workout requires a different tempo of music. **Tempo** is defined as the speed at which the music is played and is measured in beats per minute. In other words, the slower the tempo, or speed, of the song, the fewer beats per minute will occur.

The warm-up, stretch, low-impact, and cool-down routines require moderate or walking-paced music. This is measured at a range of 110 to 140 BPM (beats per minute). Peak aerobic routine tempos vary in range from 140 to 160 BPM. This is considered a jogging pace. Body toning and conditioning music should stay in a range of 110 to 130 BPM as this phase of the class should work at a walking pace.

Many aerobic dance records will list the BPM of the song. If a record you choose does not record the BPM, count the beats of the music as you would your pulse (10 seconds × 6, or 15 seconds × 4). The longer pulse count would be more appropriate for counting BPM; there is usually no change or slowing of beats within a song.

Music Analysis

Once you have selected the music, listen to the piece several times. When you are familiar with the music, divide it into musical sections: introduction, verse, chorus, instrumental, and ending.

Count the measures (8 beats to a measure) in each section and keep a record of the number of measures per section. Example:

Section	Measures
Introduction	4
Chorus	4
Verse	6
Chorus	4
Instrumental	8
Chorus	4
Verse	6
Chorus	4
Ending	2

Movement Selection

After analyzing the music, experiment by trying various dance steps to a musical section. Select a sequence of steps that lets the choreography move continuously and that can be altered in intensity so your target heart rate will be sustained. Remember that you can create variation in the dance steps by performing the movements in different spatial patterns and directions, by combining them with various arm patterns, or by adding accents with claps and snaps.

With your favorite music and combination of aerobic dance movements and steps, you can easily develop your own aerobic dance routine. Two complete aerobic routines are outlined below. You can alter the choreography of these sample routines by adding or deleting repetitions of the movement phrases as suitable to other musical selections.

Aerobic Dance Routine 1

Steps	Repetitions	Counts
INTRODUCTION		
1. Crossover jumping jacks	8, alternating right and left	2 each (total: 16)
2. Jump and clap	4	2 each (total: 8)
3. 3 runs and a hop-clap anywhere in the room	4	4 in combination (total: 16)
VERSE		
1. Jump-kick pattern: kick front, knee lift, kick side, kick front	4, alternating right and left	8 in combination (total: 32)
2. Jump lunge sideways with arm punches	4, alternating right and left	2 each (total: 8)
3. 3 runs and a pivot	2	4 in combination (total: 8)
4. Repeat jump lunge	4, alternating right and left	2 each (total: 8)
5. Repeat 3 runs and a pivot	2	4 in combination (total: 8)
CHORUS		
1. Scissors jumping jacks	4	2 each (total: 8)
2. 3 runs and a jump-clap, forward and backward	1	8 in combination

3. Repeat scissors jacks	4	2 each (total: 8)
4. Repeat 3 runs and a jump-clap, forward and backward	1	8 in combination
5. 3 turning walks and a clap	2, right and left	4 each (total: 8)
6. Jump and a clap	4	2 each (total: 8)
7. Repeat 3 turning walks and a clap	2, right and left	4 each (total: 8)
8. Repeat jump and a clap	4	2 each (total: 8)

Aerobic Dance Routine 2

Steps	*Repetitions*	*Counts*
INTRODUCTION		
1. Flea-hop	8	1 each (total: 8)
VERSE A		
1. Hopscotch	4, alternating right and left	2 each (total: 8)
2. 3 runs and a pivot	2	4 in combination (total: 8)
3. Jump-kick and clap under leg; jump-kick and clap over leg	4, alternating legs	4 in combination (total: 16)
4. ⎫		
5. ⎬ Repeat verse A steps 1, 2, and 3.		
6. ⎭		
CHORUS A		
1. Side leap right	3	2 each (total: 6)
and		
Jump-clap	2	1 each (total: 2)
2. Side leap left	3	2 each (total: 6)
and		
Jump-clap	2	1 each (total: 2)
3. Pony	8, alternating right and left	2 each (total: 16)
4. Repeat side leap right	3	2 each (total: 6)
and		
Jump-clap	2	1 each (total: 2)
5. Repeat side leap left	3	2 each (total: 6)
and		
Jump-clap	2	1 each (total: 2)
VERSE B		
Repeat verse A steps 1 through 6		
CHORUS B		
Repeat chorus A steps 1 through 5		

INSTRUMENTAL A

1. Flea-hop	8	1 each (total: 8)
2. Knee lift-jump-kick-jump	8, full pattern alternating right and left	4 in combination (total: 32)

VERSE C

Repeat verse A steps 1 through 6

CHORUS C

Repeat chorus A steps 1 through 5

INSTRUMENTAL B

Repeat instrumental A steps 1 and 2

ENDING

Jog in a big group circle	32	1 each (total: 32)

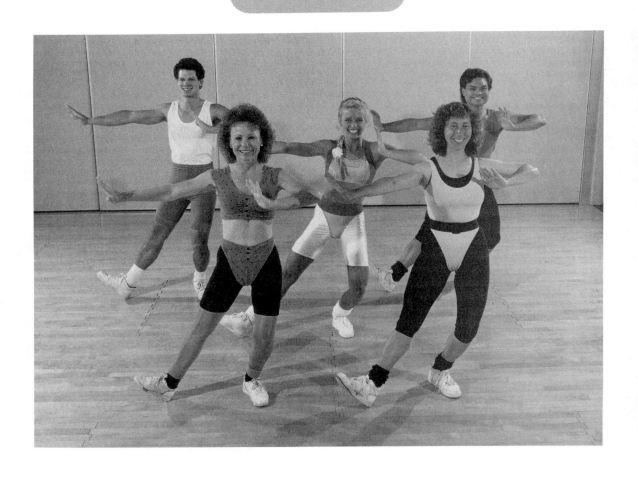

Low-Impact
and
Nonimpact Aerobics

Chapter

9

Low-impact and nonimpact movements are part of the first phase aerobics and can also be used throughout the entire aerobic segment of class. This style of aerobics is especially beneficial for people with hip, knee, and ankle problems, who often complain about the high intensity jumping and bouncing of peak aerobic dance routines. Low-impact and nonimpact aerobics provide alternatives that reduce muscular and joint stress.

In *low-impact aerobics,* one foot is always on the ground, and the shock of jumps is thus eliminated. *Nonimpact aerobics* decreases the stress even more because neither foot leaves the ground: all the movements are done by bending and straightening the knees. A nonimpact class may provide adequate exercise for the unfit or for special-needs participants, but it is generally not

strenuous enough aerobic training for the more fit individual.

Low-impact aerobics, on the other hand, can be equivalent to a high-impact aerobic workout if the routine is performed properly and the intensity of the exercise is adequate.

For an effective low-impact aerobics class, the following techniques should be applied:

1. Use full body movements and multidirectional movement patterns.
2. Move at a moderate or walking pace, using controlled movements.
3. Instead of just bending the knees, think of raising and lowering the center of gravity.
4. Emphasize movements of the legs, hips, and back; it is the use of the large muscles that elevates the heart rate.

5. Emphasize steady, rhythmic movements, and avoid jerky motions.

In low-impact aerobic routines, arm movements are large and continuous throughout the workout. Although arm movements assist in the coordination and variation of the dance steps, they do not increase oxygen consumption considerably. The use of arm or hand weights during a low-impact workout is controversial. The injury risk increases significantly with the use of weights, so the small increase in cardiovascular improvement does not outweigh the potential for injury. The leg muscles are so much larger than the arm muscles; therefore the use of large leg muscles results in higher oxygen consumption and calorie burning.

Any of the steps described in Chapter 8 can be modified to fit into a low-impact routine. As with all aerobic exercise, the heart rate should be regularly monitored and the intensity of the workout should be adjusted as necessary. Remember to keep at least one foot in contact with the floor at all times. Because of the continual use of the bent-knee position, the warm-up and cool-down should emphasize stretches specifically for the quadriceps and hamstrings. Do not bounce when performing the movements, and attempt to perform each movement through its full range of motion.

Here are some examples of how to modify aerobic dance steps:

KNEE LIFTS

Bend your supporting leg while lifting your opposite knee to your chest, to the side, or across your body. Straighten your leg as you lower your knee. You can pull your arms down toward your waist from a high position, with your elbows bending and straightening.

KICKS

Perform kicks the same as knee lifts, but extend your leg straight to the front, side, back, or across your body. You can push your arms toward the ceiling, to the sides, or in front of your body.

LUNGES

Open one leg to the front, side, or back, making sure it is bent while your other leg is straight. Then bring both legs together, knees straight. You can lift and lower your arms as you open and close your legs.

HOPSCOTCH

With your feet in a wide position, bend both knees; then straighten one leg as you lift it off the ground and bend it behind your supporting leg. You can swing your arms high toward your supporting leg or in a complete circle.

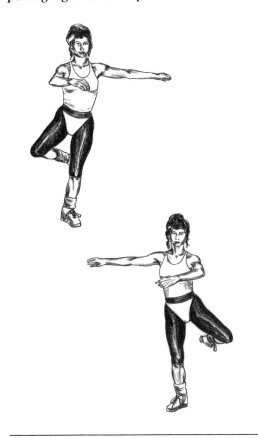

Hopscotch

JOGGING

Instead of jogging, use a power walk. This is a wide-stride walk done with the knees bent. You can punch your arms in various directions.

These modifications can be applied to any aerobic step: instead of hopping, do a kick; instead of a step-hop, do a step-kick. As in any aerobic dance class, in a low-impact class it is also important to *keep moving!*

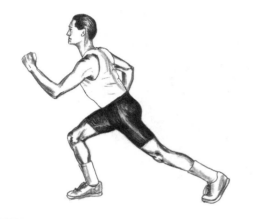

Power walk

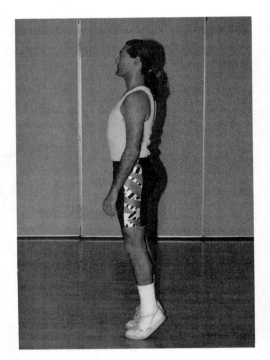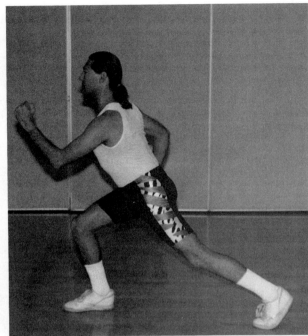

Aerobic Cool-down

Chapter

10

The aerobic cool-down follows the peak aerobic dance phase of a lesson and is designed to continue the aerobic dance movements at a lower intensity and slower pace. During the aerobic exercise phases of the workout, the heart pumps a large amount of blood to the working muscles to supply them with the oxygen needed for movement. As long as exercise continues, the muscles squeeze the veins, forcing the blood back to the heart. If exercise stops abruptly, the blood is left in the area of the working muscle. In the case of the aerobics dancer, blood may pool in the lower extremities. Because the heart has less blood to pump, blood pressure may drop, which may cause light-headedness or dizziness. However, a gradual tapering off of activity helps the muscles send the extra blood in the extremities back to the heart and brain. In addition, cool-down exercises help to prevent muscle soreness and promote faster removal of metabolic waste (4, 41).

The aerobic cool-down phase should be at least 5 minutes long for the body to have time to recover from the stress of the peak aerobic workout. Although the amount of time needed varies with each individual, the heart rate should return to 120 beats per minute or below and sweating should be reduced by the end of the aerobic cool-down phase (28). The transition from the peak aerobic workout to the aerobic cool-down phase is accomplished by gradually diminishing the intensity of the exercise and/or slowing down locomotor movements to a walking pace. Other locomotor movements include step-touches, small lunges with simple arm movements and/or upper body exercises, low knee lifts, and pliés. Fundamentally, movements should rhythmically flex and extend the legs with small, simple motions. Arm movements should be kept below heart level. Exercises used in the warm-up and in low-impact and nonimpact routines are appropriate for the aerobic cool-down.

A sample aerobic cool-down routine is described below. Vary the counts to fit your individual needs and experiment with upper body exercises as appropriate.

Aerobic Cool-Down Routine

Steps	Repetitions	Counts
INTRODUCTION		
1. Jazz square right	2	4 each (total: 8)
2. March	16	1 each (total: 16; *note* the last 2 counts have 3 steps with the rhythm 1 and 2 to change feet)
3. Jazz square left	2	4 each (total: 8)
4. March	16	1 each (total: 16; *note* the last 2 counts have 3 steps with the rhythm 1 and 2 to change feet)
VERSE A		
1. Slide forward, alternating right and left	4	2 each (total: 8)
2. Walk backward, with backward shoulder rolls	8	1 each (total: 8)
3. Slide forward, alternating right and left	4	2 each (total: 8)
4. Walk backward, with backward shoulder rolls	8	1 each (total: 8)
5. Repeat steps 1 through 4		
CHORUS A		
1. Grapevine right; touch on count 8	1	8 each
Grapevine left; touch on count 8	1	8 each
2. Right kick-ball change	2	2 each (total: 4)
3. Right pivot turn	2	2 each (total: 4)
4. Repeat grapevine right and left		
5. Repeat kick-ball change		
6. Repeat pivot turn		
VERSE B		
Repeat verse A steps 1 through 5		
CHORUS B		
Repeat chorus A steps 1 through 5		
ENDING		
Repeat introduction steps 1 through 4		
Repeat march, lowering pace to a walk	16	1 each (total: 16)

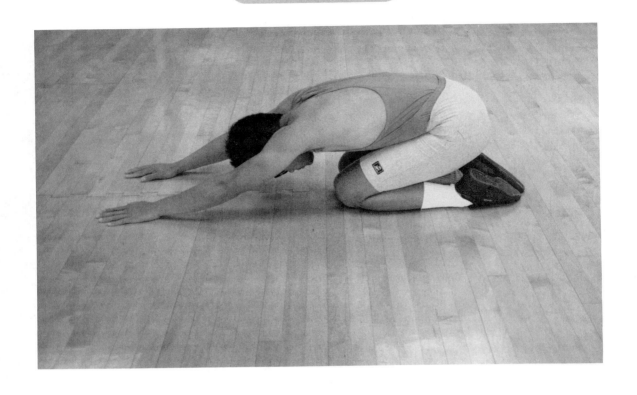

Body Toning and Conditioning

Chapter

11

The body toning and conditioning phase of the class promotes muscular strength and endurance. During this phase, equal time must be devoted to all the body's muscle groups (Figure 11–1). Body toning exercises improve the initial tone of the muscles as well as their endurance capabilities. Conditioning exercises place increased demand on muscle fibers in order to improve actual muscular strength. This session of the class is approximately 15 to 20 minutes long; the time may vary, depending on the individual instructor's format. Exercises to work specific muscle groups of the body (arms, waist, abdomen, legs, and buttocks) should be blended into the workout with smooth transitions to make the body toning and conditioning phase more enjoyable. The format emphasizes exercises for one body area at a time.

Muscle tone is the natural tension within a muscle, even when the muscle is relaxed. Muscular contraction, the tightening or shortening of a muscle, will contour and tone muscles. Muscles that are not used regularly will atrophy and look loose and flabby. Exercises that contract and strengthen the muscles give the figure shape and form. Strengthening and toning exercises are those that are performed against a force or resistance; that resistance may be in the form of pushing, pulling, or lifting your own body part or a weight.

It is important to note that even when performing an exercise for a specific muscle, other muscles will also be involved. The muscle that is the prime mover of the exercise is termed the **agonist.** The opposing muscle group that is usually stretched while the prime mover is contracted is

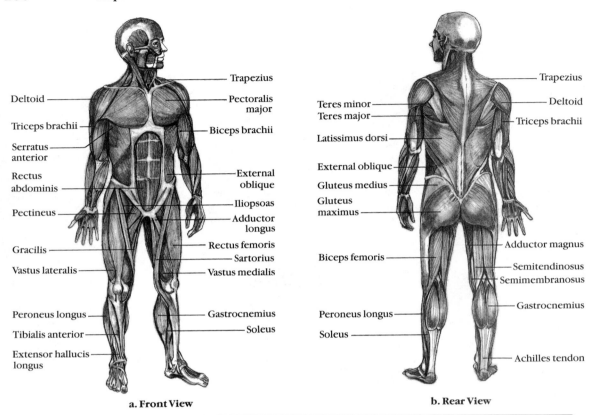

Figure 11–1 *Muscular system.*

termed the **antagonist.** Muscle groups that assist but are not the prime movers in an exercise are termed **synergists.** It is important to make each muscle an agonist and antagonist during your workout so that muscular balance is achieved.

USING WEIGHTS FOR BODY TONING

During this phase of the workout, you can use hand or ankle weights if you wish to apply overload without having to increase repetitions. Beginners should not use any weights until the workout gets easier. When it becomes necessary to add weights in order to apply overload, start with 1-pound hand weights and gradually progress to 5 pounds. Since you are not working to build bulk

but to tone, it is important to use light weights. Working up to 5-pound weights should occur over many months. Follow the rules listed below for a safe and effective workout.

1. Never swing the weights.
2. Do not squeeze the weights. Hold them firmly but gently. Holding the weights too tightly could be detrimental to your circulation.
3. Perform the exercises *slowly!* Control and tension are very important for building strength. Just going through the motions does not do the job; *tension* must be created in the muscle in order to build strength.

4. Work until the muscle is fatigued, but stop before it is in pain.
5. Perform exercises for the large muscle groups (for example, the deltoids and pectorals) before exercising the smaller muscle groups (for example, the biceps and triceps).
6. Perform 8 to 16 repetitions of an exercise before going on to a new exercise. Do a series of 3 or 4 different exercises for different muscle groups and then come back and repeat the series 2 or 3 more times.
7. Work the muscle group as well as its opposing muscle group (for example, hamstring and then quadricep or bicep and then tricep).
8. Allow a 1-minute rest of one muscle group before doing another exercise for that same group. For example, if you do an exercise for the biceps, do one next for the triceps before going back to a bicep exercise. Muscles need a rest after reaching fatigue.
9. Never hold your breath when performing any of the exercises. Breathe easily and naturally with each movement.
10. Remember to start with light weights, and always perform with proper technique.

EXERCISE EVALUATION

As you progress through the body toning and conditioning exercises introduced in this chapter, you may want to refer to Figure 11–1 to review which muscle group you are using and where it is located. In addition, it is important to evaluate each exercise you perform so that you get the maximum benefits and achieve your desired goal. The exercises in this book have been evaluated for general safety, but since each one of us is unique, it is important that each exercise work specifically for you. To evaluate each exercise, answer the five following questions.

1. What is the purpose of this exercise? Is it abdominal strength? hamstring flexibility? and so on.
2. How effective is this exercise in meeting that purpose? Am I really working my abdominals when I do a curl up?

3. Are there risks involved in performing this exercise? Does my lower back receive too much pressure? Is this exercise safe on my knee joints?
4. Can I perform this exercise with proper technique? Are my hamstrings too tight for this exercise? Do I hyperextend my back on this exercise?
5. Do I need to modify this exercise? Are my abdominals too weak for this exercise? Can I perform this exercise halfway and still receive the benefits?

To complement the strengthening exercises, flexibility exercises are included in the body toning and conditioning phase of the workout. These exercises should complement the toning and conditioning exercises by stretching previously worked muscles. For maximum flexibility, the muscles must be stretched and worked through a full range of motion. Stretching exercises may include any of those described in Chapters 7 and 12. The combination of strengthening and stretching exercises during this phase of the aerobic workout is the ideal format for improving muscle tone and aesthetic appearance.

BODY TONING AND CONDITIONING EXERCISES

Arms

Major Muscle Groups

Triceps brachii
Trapezius
Biceps brachii
Deltoid

SKY REACH

This exercise works the triceps, deltoids, and trapezius muscles. In a standing position with your feet shoulder width apart, reach both your arms upward, with your wrists flexed. Bend your elbows, keeping your arms over your head and your wrists flexed, and then straighten your arms in a pulsing motion, repeating the sky reach several times. You can also perform the sky reach by alternating arm reaches.

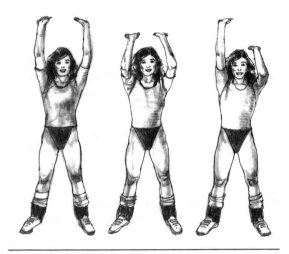

Sky reach

--- **PRECAUTION** ---

Make sure to bend your knees and contract your abdominal muscles to reduce the stress on the lower back.

ARM SCISSORS

In a standing position with your feet shoulder width apart, extend your arms forward from your chest and at shoulder height, with your palms down. "Scissor" your arms by alternately crossing one arm over the other. To exercise all muscles of the arms, vary the position of your palms: palms up, palms in, palms out. This exercise works the pectorals and deltoids.

ARM CIRCLES

In a standing position with your feet shoulder width apart, extend your arms out to the sides at shoulder height, with your palms down. Rotate your arms forward in circular motions, progressing from small to larger circles. Reverse the circular direction. You can also perform arm circles with your palms up, out, or your wrists flexed or hands held in a fist. This exercise works the deltoid and trapezius muscles.

--- **PRECAUTION** ---

In the first three exercises described, be sure to keep the head and back in proper alignment.

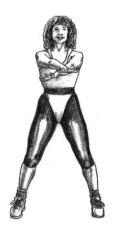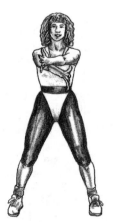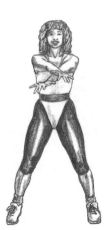

Arm scissors

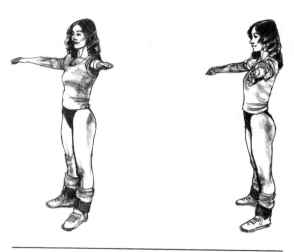

Arm circles

BICEP CURL

Stand in proper alignment, with your feet shoulder width apart and your knees slightly bent. Begin with your arms in an extended position at your sides, with your hands fisted. Bend your arms at the elbows until your hands come near your shoulders. Keep your elbows in contact with your waist. Return to the starting position.

PRECAUTIONS

- Keep your upper arms and elbows close to your sides.
- Move your lower arms only.

UPRIGHT ROW

Stand in proper alignment, with your feet shoulder width apart and your knees slightly bent. Extend your arms downward in front of your body with your hands fisted or grasping weights about a hand's width apart and facing your body. Pull your hands up your chest until they reach your chin, your elbows extending out away from your body and, at the top of the movement, in an upward position. Slowly return to the starting position. This exercise works the deltoids, biceps, and trapezius muscles.

PRECAUTIONS

- Keep your hands close to your body.
- Contract your abdominal muscles to avoid any lower back pressure.
- Do not elevate your shoulders.

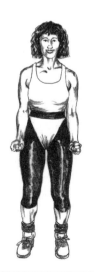
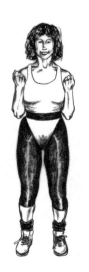

Bicep curl

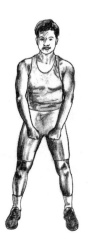
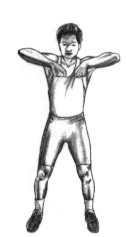

Upright row

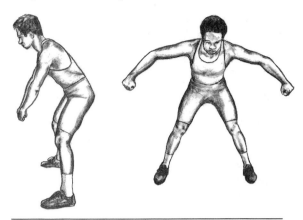

Upper back fly

UPPER BACK FLY

Start in a wide, parallel stance, leaning forward, with your torso diagonal to the floor and your knees bent. Keep your focus toward the floor. Your arms should be straight or slightly bent, hanging from the shoulders, with your hands fisted. Open your arms to the sides and then return them to the starting position. Repeat several times, slowly and with resistance. This exercise works the trapezius and rhomboid muscles.

——— PRECAUTION ———

Be sure to lean your torso forward and bend your knees.

TRICEP KICKBACK

Bend over at your waist until your upper torso is diagonal to the floor, with your feet shoulder width apart and your knees slightly bent. Keep your upper arms and elbows close to your sides. With your fisted palms facing each other, bend your lower arms up at a 45-degree angle to the upper arms. Then extend both arms behind your back until your elbows are straight. Return to the starting position.

——— PRECAUTIONS ———

- Bend your knees so there is no pressure on the back. If back pain occurs, stop the exercise.
- Keep your body stationary and only move your lower arms.

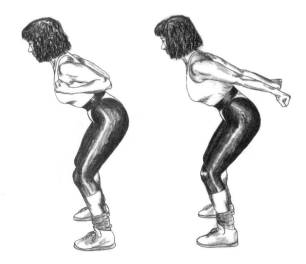

Tricep kickback

FORWARD ARM RAISE

Start in the same position as the bicep curl, but hold your arms in front of your thighs, fists facing inward. Lift your arms forward until they reach shoulder height, then return them to the starting position. This exercise develops the anterior aspect of the deltoid muscle.

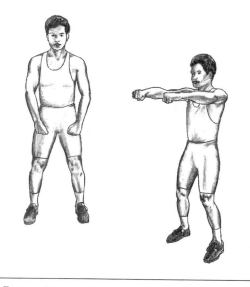

Forward arm raise

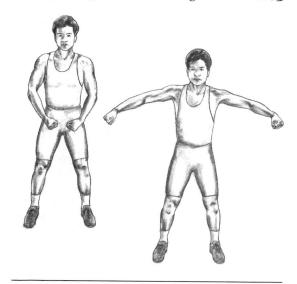

Side lateral raise

SIDE LATERAL RAISE

Start in the same position as the bicep curl, but hold your arms at your sides with your fists facing inward and your elbows slightly bent. Lift your arms out to the sides until they reach shoulder height, then return to the starting position. This exercise develops the deltoid muscle.

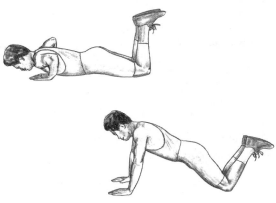

——— PRECAUTION ———

Do not lift your arms above shoulder height as this may injure the shoulders.

Modified push-up

Chest, Rib Cage, and Waist

Major Muscle Groups

Pectoralis major
Pectoralis minor (deep muscle)
Serratus anterior
Trapezius
External oblique
Teres: major and minor

Chest

MODIFIED PUSH-UP

Lie prone on the floor. Place your hands under your shoulders, with your fingers facing forward. Keep your feet together, legs bent at your knees. Keep your body in a straight plane from your knees to your head as you push your upper body off the floor until both your arms are completely straight. Lower your body back to the floor, maintaining a straight plane. Repeat the modified push-up several times. This exercise works the triceps and the pectorals.

PUSH-UP

Lie prone on the floor. Place your hands under your shoulders, with your fingers facing forward. Keep your feet together and flexed, with your body weight on the balls of your feet. Keep your body straight, abdominals and hip muscles contracted, as you push up until both your arms are straight. Lower your body halfway to the floor by bending your elbows, keeping your weight equally distributed on your hands and the balls of your feet. Repeat the push-up several times. This exercise strengthens the triceps and pectorals.

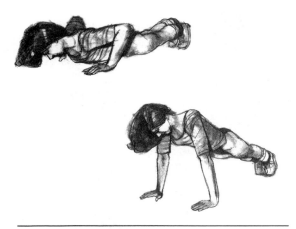

Push-up

PRECAUTIONS

- To prevent placing undue strain on the vertebrae of your lower back, do not let your lower back arch.
- Do not raise your buttocks to dip your chin.
- Do not allow your hips to sag.
- Avoid locking your elbows at the top of the exercise.
- If this exercise is too difficult, just lower your body a few inches. Do not attempt to go all the way unless you can perform the push-up correctly. Gradually build up your strength.

ARM CHEST CROSS

Stand with your feet shoulder width apart, arms extended to the sides and at shoulder height, with your palms down. Crisscross your arms in front of your body at waist height. Open your arms out to your sides. Repeat crisscrossing your arms in front of your body, progressively raising your arms until they crisscross above your head. Then continue crisscrossing your arms, lowering them back to waist level. This exercise works the deltoid and pectoral muscles.

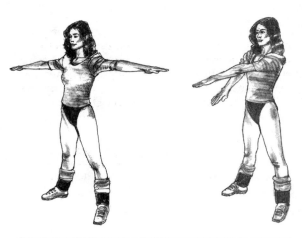

Arm chest cross

PRECAUTION

Keep your arms tight, but do not lock your elbows.

PECTORAL PRESS

Stand with your feet shoulder width apart and your knees slightly bent. Bring your arms out to your sides below shoulder height and bend your elbows, with your forearms pointing upward and your hands fisted inward. Bring your arms together in front of your body until your elbows touch. Return slowly to the starting position.

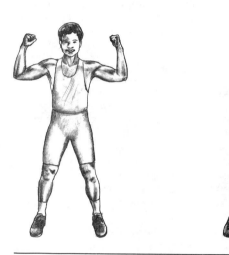

Pectoral press

Rib Cage and Waist

WAIST BEND

Stand with your feet shoulder width apart and extend your arms sideways and at shoulder height. Bend your upper body to your left, keeping your lower body stationary. Your right arm reaches overhead while your left hand rests on your left thigh for support. Repeat to the other side.

SIDE PULL

Stand with your feet shoulder width apart, with your hands crossed at your wrists in front of your body at chest height. Bend sideways to your right as your right arm reaches down and out to the right while your left elbow bends and lifts up, higher than your left shoulder. Return to the starting position. Repeat several times on both sides of your body. This exercise tones the oblique abdominals.

PRECAUTIONS

- In both exercises, make sure to bend your knees to prevent placing pressure on the lower back.
- Do not lean forward, but bend directly to the side.

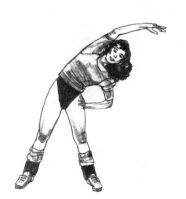

Waist bend

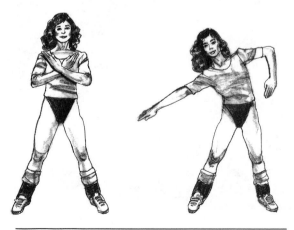

Side pull

Abdomen

Major Muscle Groups
Obliques: external and internal
Rectus abdominis
Iliopsoas

HALF SIT-UP

Lie on your back, clasp your hands behind your head, and keep your elbows back. Bend your knees, placing the soles of your feet firmly on the floor. Take a deep breath. Exhale and then contract your abdominals and press your lower back to the floor as you sit up halfway, lifting your head and shoulders off the floor. Release the contraction and lower yourself to the floor.

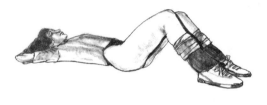

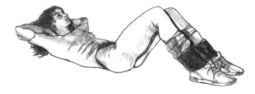

Half sit-up

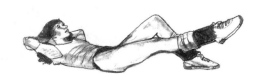

One-leg straight half sit-up

ONE-LEG STRAIGHT HALF SIT-UP

Begin in the same position as the half sit-up. Lift one leg, straight, off the floor. Proceed with the half sit-up. Repeat the exercise, lifting your other leg off the floor.

TWO-LEG HALF SIT-UP

Lie on your back, clasp your hands behind your head, and keep your elbows back. Lift both your legs, with your knees bent and feet crossed, off the floor. Proceed with the half sit-up.

————————— **PRECAUTIONS** —————————

- To reduce the possible use of the lower back muscles, it is important in all half sit-up positions to press down on your abdominals, to keep your sacrum on the floor before lifting your shoulders.
- When performing all half sit-ups, avoid placing additional stress or strain on your neck.
- If your abdominal muscles start to quiver and/or you feel yourself lifting and jerking to get up, instead of curling your back, *stop.* Such movements indicate that the abdominal muscles are tired; work will be transferred to lower back muscles, possibly causing lower back pain.

——————— **MOVEMENT TIP** ———————

If strain is felt in the neck, cross your arms over your chest and then perform all the half sit-up exercises.

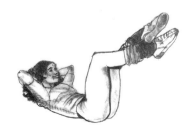

Two-leg half sit-up

ABDOMINAL CURL

Lie on your back, bend your legs, clasp your hands behind your head, and keep your elbows back. Lift your bent legs off the floor, and then lift your head and shoulders off the floor until your elbows touch your knees. Release your torso slightly away from your knees, but do *not* return to the floor. Repeat the abdominal curl. Exhale with each lift, keeping your abdominal muscles contracted.

ABDOMINAL CURL-DOWN

Begin in a sitting position, with your knees bent and your feet flat on the floor. Relax your arms at the sides of your body. Slowly lower your torso to the floor by rounding your back, contracting your stomach muscles, and placing one vertebra at a time on the floor. End in a lying position.

———— **PRECAUTION** ————

Do not let your lower back arch off the floor.

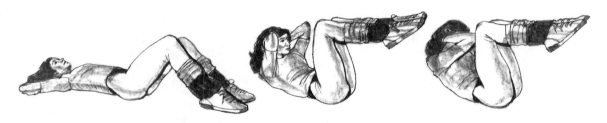

Abdominal curl

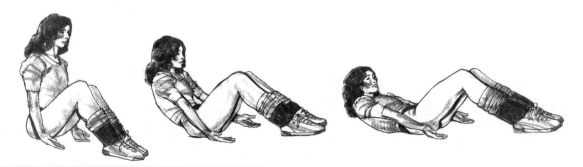

Abdominal curl-down

Hips and Buttocks

Major Muscle Groups

Gluteus maximus
Hamstrings
Iliopsoas

STARTING POSITION FOR THE LEG LIFT EXERCISES

On your hands and knees, lift one leg so that it extends straight behind you, at hip level. Lower your head by bending your elbows and leaning forward, placing your body weight over your forearms.

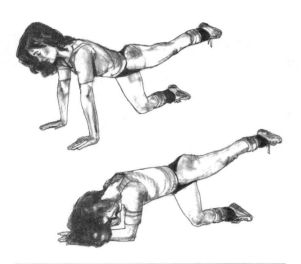

Starting position for leg lift exercises

STRAIGHT LEG LIFT

From the starting position, lift your leg up several inches, and then lower it to hip level. Repeat the exercise on your other leg. This exercise strengthens the gluteus maximus.

BENT LEG LIFT AND EXTENSION

From the starting position, bring the knee of your extended leg into your chest, and then extend your leg behind you, returning your leg to hip level. Repeat the exercise with your other leg. This exercise strengthens the gluteus maximus.

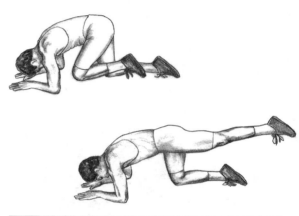

Bent leg lift and extension

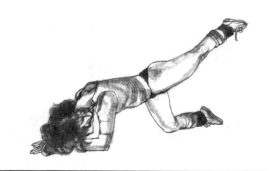

Straight leg lift

BENT-KNEE LEG LIFT

From the starting position, bend the knee of your lifted leg with your foot flexed (the sole of your foot faces the ceiling). Lift your leg in this position several inches; then lower it to hip level. Repeat on your other leg. This exercise strengthens the hamstrings and gluteus maximus.

———— PRECAUTIONS ————

- Keep your back straight by contracting your abdominal muscles to avoid placing stress or strain on your lower back.
- Do *not* lift your leg above hip level when you are on your hands and knees. By lowering your head and shifting your body weight to your forearms, you can raise your leg without tilting your pelvis or placing stress on the lumbar disk.
- Keep your hips level. Avoid turning the working hip out.

———— MOVEMENT TIP ————

All of the leg lift exercises can be performed in a standing position, facing a wall or a ballet barre.

Back

Major Muscle Groups

Serratus posterior inferior (deep muscle)
Latissimus dorsi
Erector spinae (deep muscle)
Quadratus lumborum (deep muscle)

CAT STRETCH

Begin on your hands and knees. Contract your rib cage and stomach; keep your head down. Curve your spine and hold this position for 10 seconds. Return your chest and back to a neutral position before repeating the exercise. To achieve maximum results, it is important to contract your abdominal muscles. This exercise strengthens the back musculature.

———— PRECAUTIONS ————

- Do not arch your lower back or sag in your abdominal region in the starting position.
- Do not lock your elbows.

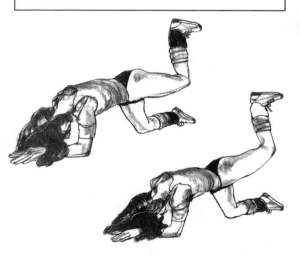

Bent-knee leg lift

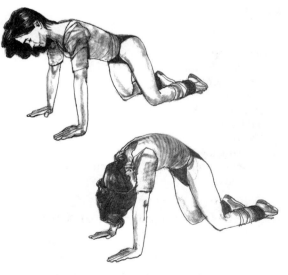

Cat stretch

ARM AND LEG LIFT

Lie prone on the floor; lift your opposite arm and leg off the floor simultaneously. Hold for a few seconds and then release. This will develop strength in both the upper and lower back.

MOVEMENT TIPS

- Always work the opposite arm and leg.
- Move slowly and with control.

CROSSOVER

Lie on your right side, your body lying flat on the floor, with your right arm extended over your head. Bend your right knee so that your thigh is in line with your torso. Raise your left leg up with your foot flexed; then lower your leg at a comfortable angle in front of you to 3 inches above the floor. Continue to lift and lower your leg in this position with your leg slightly forward. Keep your hips square (not rolling forward or backward) throughout the exercise. Reverse the crossover to your opposite side. This exercise works the abductor muscles.

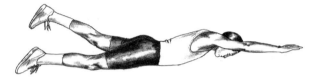

Arm and leg lift

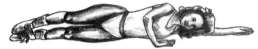

Thighs

Major Muscle Groups

Hamstrings
   Biceps femoris
   Semimembranosus
   Semitendinosus
Quadriceps femoris
   Rectus femoris
   Vastus lateralis
   Vastus medialis
   Vastus intermedius (deep muscle)
Sartorius

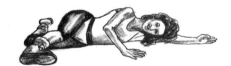

Medial Thigh Muscles

Adductors: brevis (deep muscle), longus, and
   magnus
Gracilis
Pectineus
Abductors: gluteus medius and minimus

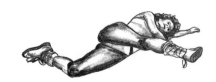

Crossover

SIDE THIGH LIFT

Lie on your right side, with your right arm extended flat along the floor. Bend your right knee so that your knee and thigh remain in line with your torso. Keeping your left leg straight with your foot flexed, toes and knee facing forward, lift your leg 1 to 2 feet off the floor. (By keeping your knee and foot facing forward, you cannot lift your leg very high. Avoid turning your knee and foot up toward the ceiling.) Continue to lift and lower your leg in this position. Reverse the side thigh lift to your opposite side. This exercise works the abductor muscles.

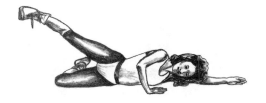

Side thigh lift

INNER THIGH LIFT

Lie on your right side, with your right arm extended flat along the floor. Bend your left knee, and place your left foot flat on the floor behind your right knee. Keeping your right leg straight with your foot flexed, toes and knee facing forward, lift your right leg as high as possible. Repeat the exercise several times. Reverse the inner thigh lift to your opposite side. This exercise works the adductor muscle group.

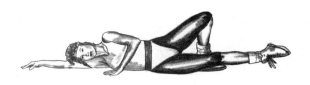

Inner thigh lift

———— PRECAUTIONS ————

- In all side thigh lift exercises, do not roll your pelvis toward your back. Stay supported directly on your side. Think of pressing your hip bones forward.
- Do not raise your leg higher than 45 degrees off the ground.

INNER THIGH BUTTERFLY

Lie on your back with your knees bent, your feet apart, the soles of your feet firmly on the floor, and your hips lifted slightly off the floor. Close your knees, pressing your inner thighs together. Separate your knees approximately 12 inches. Do not let the soles of your feet lift off the floor. Repeat the close-open motion several times. This exercise works the adductor muscle group as well as the gluteus maximus.

———— PRECAUTIONS ————

- Do not let your lower back lift off the floor.
- Do not hold your breath.

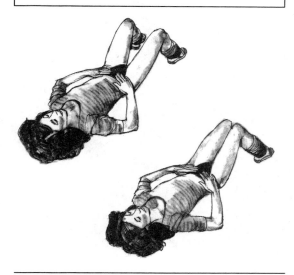

Inner thigh butterfly

FRONT THIGH LIFT

Start in a sitting position, with your legs straight forward and your feet flexed. Lift one leg slightly off the floor (2 to 3 inches). From this position, lift your leg up and down in a pulsing motion several times. Reverse the front thigh lift to your opposite leg. This exercise works the quadricep muscles.

———— PRECAUTIONS ————

- Keep your back erect.
- Do not lock your knees.

PLIÉ

Start with your feet shoulder width apart and turned out from the hip joints about 45 to 60 degrees. Keep your heels on the ground and your back and neck erect. Bend your knees as low as you can in this position. Return to the starting position by squeezing the inner thighs together. This exercise is taken from ballet and is excellent for building inner thigh, buttocks, and back strength.

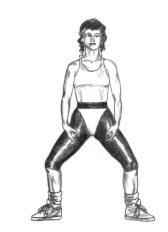

Plié

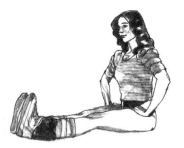

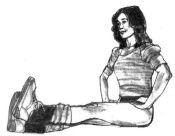

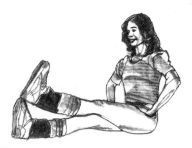

Front thigh lift

———— PRECAUTIONS ————

- Do not bend at your waist.
- Make sure your knees go out over your toes.
- This exercise can be done in conjunction with upper body exercises.
- Do not allow your buttocks to protrude. Keep them in line with your spine and maintain your pelvis in a neutral position.

SQUAT

Start with your feet about shoulder width apart and in a parallel position. You can place your hands on your shoulders. Pitch your head and torso forward as if you were going to sit in a chair. Keep your head up and your back in a straight line as you lower your buttocks until your thighs are parallel to the floor. Pause and then return to the starting position. This exercise strengthens the quadriceps, hamstrings, and the gluteus maximus.

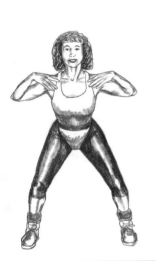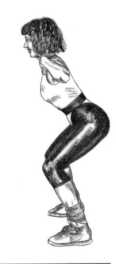

Squat

PRECAUTIONS

- Do not round your back during this exercise. Keep it elongated.
- Keep your knees in line with your toes.

MOVEMENT TIP

When performing the squat, simultaneously do one of the upper body exercises described. For example, you can perform a squat as you do an upright row or pectoral press. This will save time and work two groups of muscles at once.

LUNGE

Begin with your feet shoulder width apart and your hands resting on your shoulders. Lunge forward on your right foot until your thigh is almost parallel to the floor, your left knee still in line with your left ankle. Return to the starting position, using the buttocks muscles to push off the floor. Repeat 8 to 16 repetitions on one leg before repeating on the other side, or alternate every time. Lunges are an excellent exercise for the quadriceps, gluteus maximus, and, to a lesser extent, the calf and lower back muscles.

PRECAUTIONS

- Keep your back and neck as straight as possible.
- Be sure your forward knee stays in line with your ankle and is perpendicular to the floor.
- Contract the abdominals to relieve pressure on your knees and lower back.
- This exercise is not recommended for individuals with knee problems.

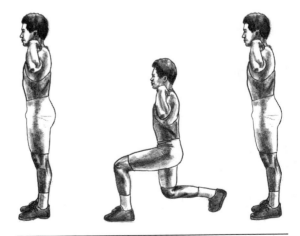

Lunge

Lower Legs and Ankles

Major Muscle Groups

Gastrocnemius
Peroneus: brevis (deep muscle) and longus
Tibialis: anterior and posterior (deep muscle)
Soleus

Flexors and Extensors of the Toes

Extensor digitorum longus (deep muscle)
Flexor digitorum longus (deep muscle)
Extensor hallucis longus
Flexor hallucis longus (deep muscle)
Flexor digitorum brevis (deep muscle)
Abductor hallucis (deep muscle)
Adductor hallucis (deep muscle)

HEEL RAISE

Stand with your feet in a parallel position about shoulder width apart. Rise onto the balls of your feet as far as possible, and then slowly lower to the starting position. This exercise will develop the gastrocnemius and achilles tendon.

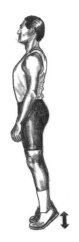

Heel raise

FOOT LIFT

Stand with your back against a wall, with your feet about 12 inches from the wall. Raise and lower your feet several times. You can raise your feet together and/or alternate them (27).

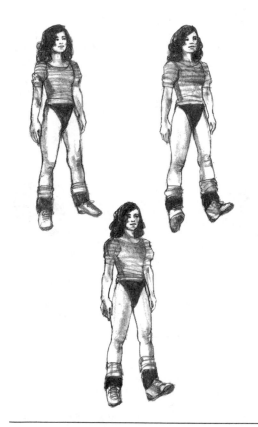

Foot lift

FOOT PRESS

Sit on the floor with your legs straight out in front of you. Have a partner sit in front of your legs and grasp both your feet; your toes should be pointed. Your partner applies downward pressure as you try to flex your ankle. Work through the full range of motion. Do not bend your knees. Repeat the exercise several times (27).

BODY TONING AND CONDITIONING ROUTINES

Body toning and conditioning routines are made up of many of the exercises in this chapter combined with stretching exercises. Routines should involve all body parts, with smooth transitions from one exercise to the next. Two sample routines are described below. (Stretching exercises, which follow the body toning and conditioning phase, are described in Chapter 12.) You may vary your performance of the repetitions and/or counts of each exercise to fit your individual needs.

Floor Body Toning Routine

Exercise	*Repetitions*	*Counts*
Push-up	16	2 up, 2 down
Chest stretch (see Chapter 7)	1	16
Side thigh lift	16	1 up, 1 down
Inner thigh lift	16	1 up, 1 down
Pretzel (see Chapter 12)	1 right, 1 left	16 each side
Butterfly stretch	1	16
Straight leg lift	16 right, 16 left	1 up, 1 down
Bent-knee leg lift	16 right, 16 left	1 up, 1 down
Buttocks to heels reach stretch (see Chapter 12)	1	16
Arm and leg lift	8 right, 8 left	1 up, hold 2, 1 down
Half sit-up	16	1 up, 1 down
Two-leg half sit-up	16	1 up, 1 down
Abdominal curl	16	1 up, 1 down
Relax on your back; stretch your arms over your head	1	16

Standing Body Toning Routine

Exercise	*Repetitions*	*Counts*
Side lateral raise	12	4 up, 4 down
Forward arm raises	12	4 up, 4 down
Upright row	12	4 up, 4 down
Arm Scissors	12	8 in each position
Pectoral press	12	4 in, 4 out
Bicep curl	12	4 up, 4 down
Tricep kickback	12	4 to straighten, 4 to bend

Upper Body Stretches

Exercise	Repetitions	Counts
Elbow clasp overhead (see Chapter 12)	1	32
Chest stretch (see Chapter 7)	1	32
Lateral stretch (see Chapter 7)	1 right, 1 left	16 each side

As the standing body toning routine becomes comfortable, you should repeat one and then two more sets of all the exercises as you simultaneously perform 12 squats (4 counts to lower and 4 counts to recover), 12 lunges right, 12 lunges left, 12 squats, 12 lunges right, 12 lunges left, and stay stationary for the tricep kickback.

Above are listed upper body stretches that should be performed following the preceding routines.

As these routines become easier, apply overload by adding hand weights for the arms and ankle weights for the floor work. Place weights on the abdomen or chest to overload on the abdominal exercises.

IS IT POSSIBLE TO SPOT REDUCE?

Evidence proves that spot reducing is a claim, *not* a fact. The public has been led to believe that blubbery thighs, hips, and arms are merely cosmetic problems. People who promote spot reducing are actually reinforcing a sedentary lifestyle, which is an initial factor in bringing about weight gain and muscular degeneration in the first place.

Exercise of a particular muscle cannot decrease the number of fat cells that lie immediately around that muscle. Also, exercise does not change fat into muscle; fatty tissue and muscular tissue are *not* the same and are not interchangeable. The only way to rid your body of unsightly fat is to reduce the amount of fat or to reduce the size of existing fat tissues.

Working muscles draw their source of energy from fat all over the body. As a result of exercise, fat from all over the body is released, converted into energy, and then used by the muscles. This breakdown of fat to energy is due to the interaction of the nervous, circulatory, muscular, and endocrine systems and is the only way to rid the body of its fatty deposits.

Spot reducing exercises *seem* to work for two reasons. First, we tend to lose fat first from the area of greatest concentration. Second, when normally unexercised, weakened muscles are exercised, the muscle beneath the fat tissue is strengthened and toned. For example, a woman plagued with what appears to be fat deposits on the back of her arm may really have a weakened triceps muscle. Push-ups and arm-strengthening exercises can help strengthen and tone that muscle, firming the arm area. The circumference of that area may be reduced as a result of improved muscle tone. As a consequence, it may appear that the spot reducing exercise works.

But do not be fooled; fat cannot be rolled, shimmied, or shaken off. Saunas and rubberized sweat suits won't rid you of pounds of fat—only water! Only a comprehensive fitness program can help you evaluate your fitness and fat level and help you achieve better overall health and fitness.

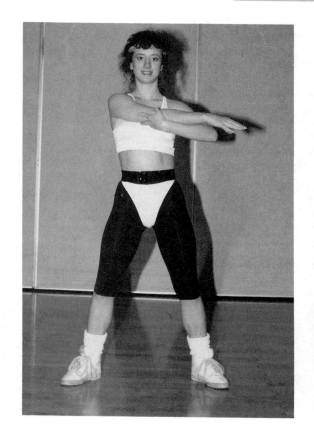
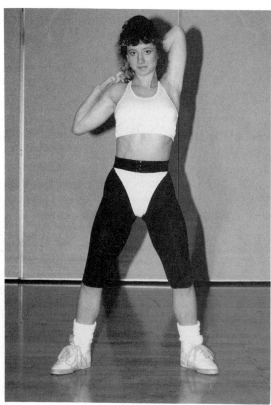

Flexibility Cool-down

Chapter

12

Just as the warm-up prepares the body for activity, flexibility stretching allows the body to prepare for rest. Stretching at this phase of the lesson is safe and effective because the muscles are warm and allow for a deeper static stretch. Remember that adequate flexibility is critical for preventing injury and minimizing soreness and fatigue. Flexibility exercises are designed to maintain and increase good joint flexibility and muscular elasticity. It is important that flexibility exercises avoid awkward body positions and that the transitions between exercises be smooth. Careless stretching and improper technique can actually result in muscle tears and damage. Proper stretching technique is extremely important for the aerobic dancer.

A long, sustained (static) stretch rather than a bouncing (ballistic) stretch is best. Muscles have a stretch reflex; when you bounce, the reflex causes the muscles to react by tightening rather than by stretching.

PROPER STRETCHING TECHNIQUES

When you are stretching, go to the point of mild tension. Relax in this position, and hold the stretch for 10 to 30 seconds. Release your position, and repeat the stretch. Before stretching a specific muscle, contract the opposing muscle. The reciprocal stretch exercise technique involves an isometric contraction of agonist muscles followed by a passive stretch of antagonist muscles of the same muscle group. For example, contract the quadriceps and then follow with a passive stretch of the hamstrings.

Always perform the exercises with proper body alignment. Two key areas of concern are the lower back and knees. Avoid holding your breath during any phase of an exercise; not breathing indicates a lack of relaxation. If your body vibrates or shakes during a stretch, ease up—you cannot relax if you are straining.

As you progress in the stretching exercises, keep in mind that flexibility is highly individual. Not all stretching exercises are appropriate for all people. Flexibility varies widely among people and also among the joints and muscles within each individual. Anatomical abnormalities and/or improperly performing an exercise can result in injury. If you perform an exercise correctly but experience abnormal pain, discontinue that particular exercise and seek professional advice regarding the problem.

The following section describes specific stretching exercises and their proper techniques. The exercises described in Chapter 7 can also be used during the cool-down phase of class.

STRETCHING EXERCISES

Neck

HEAD RAISE

Lie on your back with your knees bent, the soles of your feet on the floor, and your hands clasped behind your head. Lift your head off the floor, pulling your chin toward your chest. Hold this position for 4 counts, and then lower your head in 4 counts, stretching your neck away from your spine as your head releases to the floor.

PRECAUTIONS ————

- Do not force your neck to flex and hyperextend while exercising. Added momentum and quick, abrupt movements can damage neck ligaments.
- Do not overbend your neck by bearing your body weight in this area; doing so places additional pressure on the disks and bones (35).

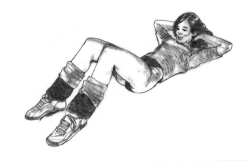

Head raise

Warm-up Exercise That Can Be Used in the Cool-down

Neck isolations

Chest, Rib Cage, Waist, and Arms

HAND CLASP OVER HEAD

Clasp your hands above your head and press your palms toward the ceiling, stretching your arms up and back. In this position, stretch to one side. Repeat the exercise to the other side. You can perform this exercise while standing, sitting, or kneeling. If standing, keep your knees relaxed.

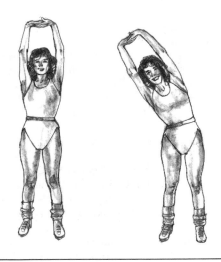

Hand clasp over head

ELBOW CLASP OVER HEAD

Cross your arms in front of your body and hold your elbows with your hands. Raise your elbows overhead and pull back. For extra stretch, pull one elbow at a time. You can perform this exercise while standing, sitting, or kneeling.

LUNGE WITH OVERHEAD OPPOSITION PULL

Start by standing in a straddle position, with your arms overhead, your left hand grasping your right wrist. Lunge onto your right leg, bending sideways at your waist to the left as your left arm pulls your right arm straight over your head. Reverse the stretch to the opposite side.

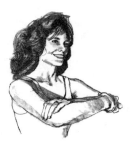

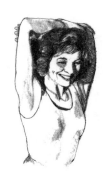

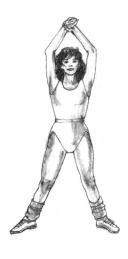

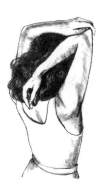

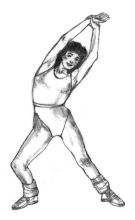

Elbow clasp over head

Lunge with overhead opposition pull

DELTOID ACROSS-CHEST OPPOSITION PULL

Start by standing in a straddle position, with your arms straight out in front of your chest, your left hand grasping your right wrist. Lunge onto your right leg, and pull your right arm across your chest to the left side of your body. Reverse the stretch to the opposite side. This is also an excellent stretch for the triceps.

SHOULDER PRESS

Stand in a straddle position, with your knees bent over your toes. Bend forward at your hips and place your hands on your knees to support your upper body. Once you are in this position, slowly press one shoulder as far forward as possible. Hold the stretch, and then repeat it on the other side. This exercise not only stretches the shoulder girdle, but also is beneficial in relieving compression in the lower back.

PRECAUTIONS

- Be sure to contract your abdominal muscles.
- Keep your knees in line with your toes.
- Keep your lower back in a rounded position.

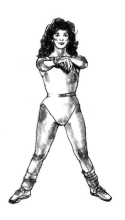

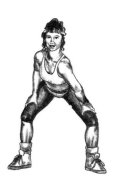

Shoulder press

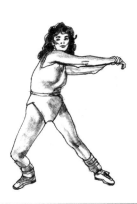

Deltoid across-chest opposition pull

Warm-up Exercises That Can Be Used in the Cool-down

Across-the-body stretch
Upper back stretches
Chest stretch
Shoulder circles
Shoulder shrugs
Lateral stretch
Reach stretch

Back

SPINAL ROTATION

Lie on your back, with your knees bent to your chest and your arms extended out to the sides at shoulder height. Drop your knees to the right, and look at your left hand. Keep both shoulders on the floor, and relax in this position. Repeat on the other side. For individuals with back problems, keep your feet on the floor while lowering your knees to the side.

——— **PRECAUTIONS** ———

- Do not arch your back.
- Do not hold your breath.

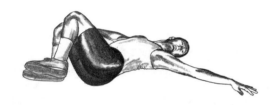

Spinal rotation

BUTTOCKS TO HEELS REACH STRETCH

Kneeling on the floor, keep your buttocks as close to your heels as possible. Relax your upper body over your thighs, and reach your arms forward along the floor. This exercise is excellent for relieving stress in the lower back as well as stretching the chest, shoulder, and tricep muscles.

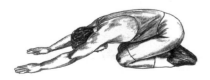

Buttocks to heels reach stretch

Warm-up Exercises That Can Be Used in the Cool-down

Upper back stretches
Knee lift stretch
Lower back alignment exercises from Chapter 6

Thighs

Warm-up Exercises That Can Be Used in the Cool-down

Knee lift stretch
Runner lunge
Quadricep stretch
Hamstring stretch
Wide and deep knee bend

Legs and Groin

FOOT-TO-GROIN STRADDLE STRETCH

Bend your right leg so that your right foot touches your groin. Relax the trunk of your body over your left leg. Repeat the stretch on your right leg.

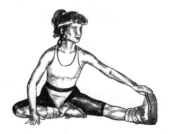

Foot-to-groin straddle stretch

———————— **PRECAUTION** ————————

A groin stretch, commonly called the *hurdler's stretch* (one leg is bent so that the foot touches the buttocks while the trunk of the body stretches forward over an extended leg), can gradually stretch the ligaments on the inside of the knee (medial collateral ligament) and the tissue of the groin, causing painful fascial groin pulls.

STARTING POSITION FOR STRADDLE STRETCH

Sitting with your back straight, open your legs as wide as possible to a straddle position. Your hips will remain on the floor, and your knees will face the ceiling on the toward-the-leg straddle stretch and straddle side stretch.

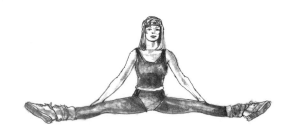

Starting position for straddle stretch

———————— **PRECAUTIONS** ————————

- Do not let your legs roll forward. Keep your knees rotated toward the ceiling.
- Keep your knees relaxed.
- Do not allow either buttock to lift from the floor.

TOWARD-THE-LEG STRADDLE STRETCH

Twist from your waist as far as possible toward your right leg. Reach toward your right ankle with both your hands, gently pulling your chest toward your right leg. To help keep your back straight, imagine putting your chin on your shin. Repeat the stretch to your left leg.

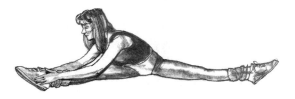

Toward-the-leg straddle stretch

STRADDLE SIDE STRETCH

Place your right arm from your elbow to your palm on the floor, either inside or outside your right leg. Your left arm reaches overhead while you are stretching your right leg. Reverse the stretch toward your left leg.

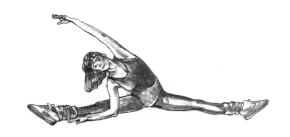

Straddle side stretch

Warm-up Exercises That Can Be Used in the Cool-down

Runner lunge
Side lunge
Side lunge to the floor
Knee lift stretch

Hips

INDIAN SIT GLUTEAL STRETCH

Sitting with your back straight, cross your legs Indian style. Keep both your hips in contact with the floor. Reverse the cross of your legs to stretch both hips equally. Isolations, rib cage, waist, and arm movements may be performed in this position.

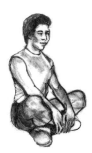

Indian sit gluteal stretch

BUTTERFLY STRETCH

Sitting with your back straight, bring the soles of your feet together, with your knees bent. Hold your ankles, and press your pelvic girdle forward, keeping your back straight. Gently press your knees toward the floor to increase the flexibility of your hip joints.

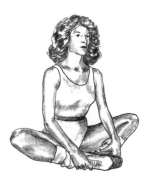

Butterfly stretch

PRETZEL

Sitting with your back straight, cross your legs Indian style. Lift your right leg and place your right foot on the outside of your left thigh, keeping all five toes in contact with the floor. Keep your back straight, and pull your right knee toward your chest with your left arm while pressing your hip toward the floor. Reverse the stretch to your left leg.

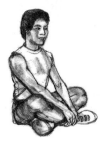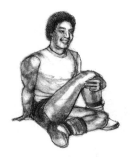

Pretzel

GLUTEAL STRETCH

Lying on your back, start with your knees bent and the soles of your feet on the ground. Cross your right ankle onto your left thigh. Pull your knees to your chest by grasping your left thigh. Repeat this stretch on your left leg.

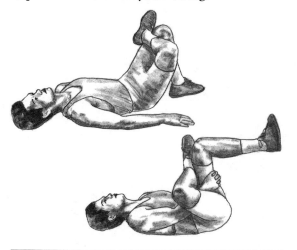

Gluteal stretch

Warm-up Exercises That Can Be Used in the Cool-down

Runner lunge
Side lunge
Knee lift stretch

Abdomen

ABDOMINAL STRETCH

Lying on your back, stretch your arms overhead while stretching your legs and flexing your feet. This stretch is effective immediately after abdominal strengthening and endurance exercises.

PELVIC TILT

Lie on your back, with your knees bent, the soles of your feet on the floor, and your hands at your sides. Tightening your buttocks, lift your hips toward the ceiling, approximately 4 inches off the floor. Release the stretch, lowering your back and hips to the floor one vertebra at a time. The pelvic tilt also stretches the thigh and abdominal muscles. *Note:* The pelvic tilt may be done as a body toning exercise by advanced students who understand the body concept of tightening the gluteus and abdominal muscles to support the lower back. As a body toning and conditioning exercise, the pelvic tilt is done repeatedly in more rapid succession and works to tone and condition the gluteus muscle.

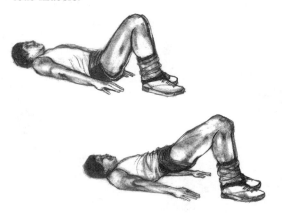

Pelvic tilt

LOW COBRA

Lying prone on the floor, place your hands on the floor near your shoulders. Keeping your elbows on the floor, lift your chest off the floor and arch your upper back. Keep your hips down and lower back relaxed. Slowly bend your arms to lower your chest to the starting position. Do several rhythmic repetitions.

──────────── **PRECAUTION** ────────────

Avoid the "swan" version (overarched lower back position) of this exercise, which places excessive hypertension in the lumbar area.

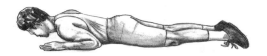

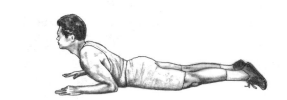

Low cobra

Lower Legs

Warm-up Exercises That Can Be Used in the Cool-down

Calf stretch
Soleus stretch
Toe tap

Ankles

ANKLE CIRCLES

Slowly circle your foot; be sure to circle in both directions. You can perform this exercise while standing or sitting.

Warm-up Exercise That Can Be Used in the Cool-down

Ankle flexion and extension

COOL-DOWN ROUTINES

Cool-down routines are made up of many of the stretches described in this chapter. The routines should flow from one stretch to the next, and all body parts should be used. A sample routine is now described; you can vary the counts to fit your individual needs.

Cool-Down Routine

Stretch	*Repetitions*	*Counts*
Gluteal stretch	1 right, 1 left	16 each
Spinal rotation	1 right, 1 left	16 each
Pelvic tilt	2	16 each
Foot-to-groin straddle stretch	1 right, 1 left	16 each
Pretzel	1 right, 1 left	16 each
Ankle circles (sitting, legs relaxed in front)	8 right, 8 left	2 each
Neck isolations (sitting Indian style)	4 right, 4 left	4 each
Hand clasp over head (sitting Indian style)	1 right, 1 left	16 each
Come to a standing position		
Shoulder press	1 right, 1 left	16 each
Lunge with overhead opposition pull	1 right, 1 left	16 each
End in proper alignment with 2 deep inhales and exhales.		

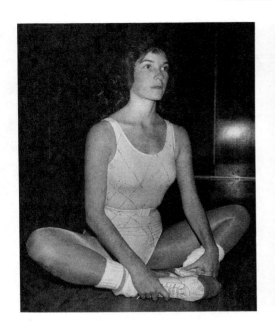
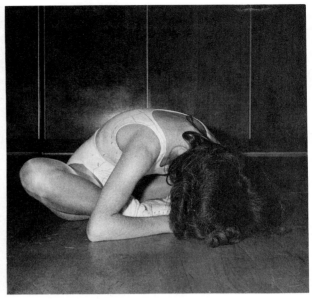

Stress and Relaxation

Chapter

13

It is impossible to live in today's world without experiencing occasional states of stress. A certain amount of stress is necessary for life to be maintained, for people to resist aggression and adapt to constantly changing external influences. Because stress is inevitable, we must learn to cope with it and to understand when stress has become distress.

Symptoms of abnormal states of stress include restlessness, lack of concentration, tension, anxiety, unreasonable irritability and depression, headaches, insomnia, nightmares, depressed appetite, or increased smoking (9). Everyone occasionally experiences one or more of these states, but it is not normal to be continually beset with them. There are many passive and active techniques to help individuals manage stress. For some of us, relaxation is a skill we must acquire. In our complex world, a life totally devoid of stress is nearly impossible, but by taking the time and making a conscious effort, we can achieve the ability to relax. To quote the poet Ovid: "What is without periods of rest will not endure."

PASSIVE RELAXATION TECHNIQUES

Passive relaxation techniques include total relaxation, meditation, and visual imagery. A quiet room with minimal distractions is necessary for following through with these mental relaxation techniques.

Total Relaxation

Lie on your back in a comfortable position. Take a deep breath, counting to 5 when you inhale;

count to 10 when you exhale. Focus your concentration on this breathing pattern, mentally dismissing all outside distractions. As you continue, begin to form a mental image of how you look when you are relaxed: Your jaw has dropped; your neck is loose; your eyes are drowsy; your legs, hips, and back are heavy. Your breathing is light and easy. Continue this exercise for at least 5 to 10 minutes to experience a state of total relaxation.

Meditation

Sit in a cross-legged position, resting your hands in your lap or on your knees. Close your eyes and totally relax all your muscles. Concentrate on a simple, single word or sound while breathing slowly and rhythmically. If your mind drifts, refocus on the word or sound. Continue thinking of that one word or sound for about 20 minutes. When you finish, sit quietly for several minutes with your eyes open. Then stand up slowly.

Visual Imagery

Lie on your back and get as comfortable as possible. Close your eyes and begin to build a serene world in your mind, such as a mountain lake with the sun shining and a warm breeze blowing. Visualize every detail of the scene, and place yourself in this environment. Continue this visualization for at least 10 minutes. Open your eyes and sit quietly for several minutes. Then stand up slowly.

ACTIVE RELAXATION TECHNIQUES

Find a warm, quiet space with as few distractions as possible. Your body must be in a relaxed position. For the sitting position, rest your hands on your thighs, with your fingers spread, head hung gently forward, and all your muscles relaxed. For the lying position, lie on a bed or the floor. Spread your legs, let your feet point away from your body, place your arms away from the sides of your body with your palms down and fingers spread. For added support, you can place a pillow or rolled towel under your neck, at the curve in your lower back, and under your knees and elbows (49). Give yourself at least 10 minutes

to complete the following exercises in a relaxed manner.

Progressive Relaxation

The goal of this technique is to achieve the sensation of complete muscular relaxation after experiencing complete muscular tension.

First lie on your back with your legs straight and your hands at the sides of your body. Relax as best as you can.

Next, contract your facial muscles by tightly closing your eyes and clenching your teeth, keeping your mouth tightly closed. Release the tension slowly to the count of 10.

Clench your fist as hard as you can and hold the position for 5 seconds and feel the tension. Feel the tension in your arm? Release the tension very slowly to the count of 10. Repeat this exercise with your other arm.

Flex your feet and tighten the quadricep muscles in each leg. Hold the tension for 5 seconds and feel the tension. Release slowly to the count of 10. Repeat this tension and relaxation process by tightening and releasing your buttock and stomach muscles.

Slow, Controlled Movements for Your Head and Torso

Slow, controlled movements or large, rhythmical, free-flowing movements also help promote relaxation. Sit on the floor or in a chair in a comfortable position so that you feel no undue muscular tension. Breathe slowly and rhythmically when performing the following movements.

Perform slow, easy neck swings; do not swing your head to the back. Now perform slow, easy shoulder circles. Next, perform slow, easy side bends with your spine, keeping your arms relaxed at your sides. Relax your spine forward and breathe easily.

Exercise can also be a tool for releasing daily tension and increasing your ability to understand stressful conditions. Although experts cannot agree about exactly how exercise works this way, various theories suggest (1) that exercise may simply be a diversion, freeing the mind from stresses that contribute to anxiety; (2) that a feeling of accomplishment (of a physical goal) is a factor; and (3) that exercise reduces muscular tension, thus inducing a state of muscular relaxation. If you exercise to help reduce stress, you must not overexercise, which will recreate a state of stress.

A properly designed aerobic program is a way to reduce levels of stress. However, the program must be within your capacity so that you are not overstressed. Your participation must not lead to staleness or chronic fatigue or cause you to become obsessive about exercise (49).

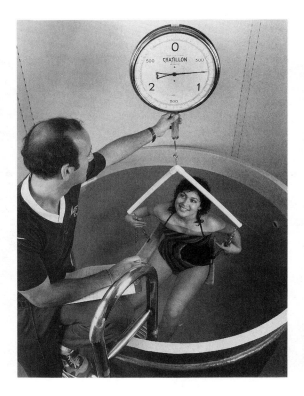
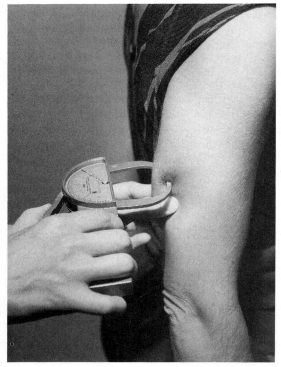

Photograph of hydrostatic tank provided by Alan Rosenberg.

Body Composition

Chapter

14

How often do we hear the common complaint, "I'm overweight"? Most people are concerned if they are "overweight," but what they should actually be concerned about is being "overfat." Too many people use scale weight to evaluate their body fitness and health, but we now know that fat can be "hidden" within the body; the scale shows no evidence of fat gain. For example, the average American adult exercises less and eats, drinks, and sits more. As a result, the muscles become less dense, less lean, less "hard." These unused muscles weigh less than they did when they were exercised, and fat begins to accumulate in the body. What used to be "muscle weight" has been exchanged for "fat weight" within the body. This helps explain why we may keep weighing the same but look heavier.

In order to understand the difference between the weight as it appears on the scale and the way the body looks, we must understand body composition. **Body composition** is generally assessed by two basic methods: (1) body fat determination, which measures the body's relative proportions of fat weight and lean body weight, and (2) **somatotyping,** which classifies the human body among three different body types.

FAT WEIGHT

There are two forms of body fat: essential fat and nonessential, or storage, fat. *Essential fat* is stored in the bone marrow, in organs like the heart, lungs, liver, spleen, kidneys, intestines, and in the liquid-rich tissues of the spinal column and brain. *Storage fat* accumulates in adipose tissue, the fatty tissues that protect the various internal organs and that are found in the subcutaneous fat deposited beneath the skin. A certain amount of storage fat in every person's body is necessary for maintaining health and good nutrition. Women and men need different amounts of essential storage fat: A healthy adult female should have approximately 20- to 25-percent body fat; a healthy adult male, 15- to 18-percent. Note that these are not necessarily "ideal" percentages; good athletes often drop below these average figures, and high-performance female athletes often have 10-percent body fat, males 7 percent. Your percentage of body fat should not become so low as to impinge on your stores of essential fat (below 10 percent for women, below 3 percent for men).

LEAN BODY WEIGHT

Lean body weight is the collective weight of the bones, muscles, ligaments and connective tissues, organs, and fluids. During adulthood, changes in lean body weight may occur primarily because the body's muscles are not receiving as much exercise. Although your life may be filled with activity, do not confuse that activity with exercise, which stresses the muscles. You need to regularly exercise your muscles to keep them lean and dense.

Three methods can be used to determine the body's percentages of fat and lean weight: (1) hydrostatic weighing, (2) skinfold measurement, and (3) the body composition analyzer.

Hydrostatic Weighing

The *hydrostatic,* or underwater immersion, *test* is a very accurate method for determining body composition. A person is weighed under water to determine body density: The more bone and muscle content the person has, the more easily the person sinks. Because fat floats, the more fat content a person has, the less the person weighs under water.

The underwater weighing technique is based on the use of Archimede's principle, which states that an object immersed in fluid loses an amount of weight in water equivalent to the weight of the fluid that is displaced. The density can be determined indirectly by measuring the change in weight when the object (person) is fully immersed (24).

Hydrostatic weighing is not as simple as it sounds and is usually unavailable to most people because it is expensive and involves sophisticated laboratory equipment. You may inquire about this technique at colleges and universities; many schools use it in their physical fitness education programs.

Skinfold Measurement

A calibrated precision instrument called a *skinfold caliper* is used to measure several predetermined sites on the body to determine the amount of body fat that lies just under the skin. The measurements we describe below—the Pollock, Schmidt, and Jackson method—are taken at three skinfold sites and provide a fat percentage based on a subject's age (see the illustrations opposite) (24).

These measurements are then computed by a formula to assess the amount of total body fat. (See the charts on pages 138 and 139.) Although this method is relatively simple as compared to hydrostatic weighing and the body composition analyzer, it is not as accurate because it gives an estimate of only body fat, not body mass. The accuracy rate is ±5 to 10 percent of body fat. Because approximately 50 percent of total body fat lies just under the skin and the skinfold test is easy to administer, the method is widely used. It is also a useful comparative test: The original body fat measurements can be compared with new measurements taken at the same sites after months of training or exercising.

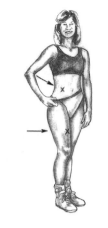

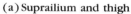

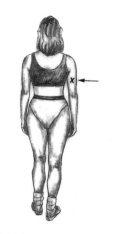

(a) Suprailium and thigh   (b) Triceps

Skinfold sites for women

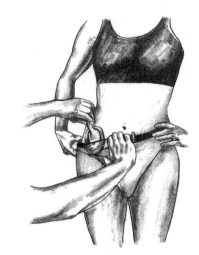

Suprailium skinfold for women: Grasp a diagonal skinfold just above the crest of the ilium, where an imaginary anterior axillary line intersects.

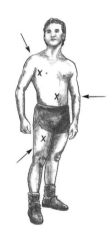

Skinfold sites for men: chest, abdomen, and thigh.

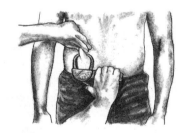

Abdominal skinfold for men: Grasp a vertical skinfold 2 to 2.5 centimeters lateral (left) of the umbilicus.

Estimating Body Fat Percentages in Women: Sum of Triceps, Suprailium, and Thigh Skinfolds

SUM OF SKINFOLDS (mm)	UNDER 22	23–27	28–32	33–37	38–42	43–47	48–52	53–57	OVER 57
23–25	9.7	9.9	10.2	10.4	10.7	10.9	11.2	11.4	11.7
26–28	11.0	11.2	11.5	11.7	12.0	12.3	12.5	12.7	13.0
29–31	12.3	12.5	12.8	13.0	13.3	13.5	13.8	14.0	14.3
32–34	13.6	13.8	14.0	14.3	14.5	14.8	15.0	15.3	15.5
35–37	14.8	15.0	15.3	15.5	15.8	16.0	16.3	16.5	16.8
38–40	16.0	16.3	16.5	16.7	17.0	17.2	17.5	17.7	18.0
41–43	17.2	17.4	17.7	17.9	18.2	18.4	18.7	18.9	19.2
44–46	18.3	18.6	18.8	19.1	19.3	19.6	19.8	20.1	20.3
47–49	19.5	19.7	20.0	20.2	20.5	20.7	21.0	21.2	21.5
50–52	20.6	20.8	21.1	21.3	21.6	21.8	22.1	22.3	22.6
53–55	21.7	21.9	22.1	22.4	22.6	22.9	23.1	23.4	23.6
56–58	22.7	23.0	23.2	23.4	23.7	23.9	24.2	24.4	24.7
59–61	23.7	24.0	24.2	24.5	24.7	25.0	25.2	25.5	25.7
62–64	24.7	25.0	25.2	25.5	25.7	26.0	26.7	26.4	26.7
65–67	25.7	25.9	26.2	26.4	26.7	26.9	27.2	27.4	27.7
68–70	26.6	26.9	27.1	27.4	27.6	27.9	28.1	28.4	28.6
71–73	27.5	27.8	28.0	28.3	28.5	28.8	29.0	29.3	29.5
74–76	28.4	28.7	28.9	29.2	29.4	29.7	29.9	30.2	30.4
77–79	29.3	29.5	29.8	30.0	30.3	31.4	31.6	31.0	31.3
80–82	30.1	30.4	30.6	30.9	31.1	31.4	31.6	31.9	32.1
83–85	30.9	31.2	31.4	31.7	31.9	32.2	32.4	32.7	32.9
86–88	31.7	32.0	32.2	32.5	32.7	32.9	33.2	33.4	33.7
89–91	32.5	32.7	33.0	33.2	33.5	33.7	33.9	34.2	34.4
92–94	33.2	33.4	33.7	33.9	34.2	34.4	34.7	34.9	35.2
95–97	33.9	34.1	34.4	34.6	34.9	35.1	35.4	35.6	35.9
98–100	34.6	34.8	35.1	35.3	35.5	35.8	36.0	36.3	36.5
101–103	35.3	35.4	35.7	35.9	36.2	36.4	36.7	36.9	37.2
104–106	35.8	36.1	36.3	36.6	36.8	37.1	37.3	37.5	37.8
107–109	36.4	36.7	36.9	37.1	37.4	37.6	37.9	38.1	38.4
110–112	37.0	37.2	37.5	37.7	38.0	38.2	38.5	38.7	38.9
113–115	37.5	37.8	38.0	38.2	38.5	38.7	39.0	39.2	39.5
116–118	38.0	38.3	38.5	38.8	39.0	39.3	39.5	39.7	40.0
119–121	38.5	38.7	39.0	39.2	39.5	39.7	40.0	40.2	40.5
122–124	39.0	39.2	39.4	39.7	39.9	40.2	40.4	40.7	40.9
125–127	39.4	39.6	39.9	40.1	40.4	40.6	40.9	41.1	41.4
128–130	39.8	40.0	40.3	40.5	40.8	41.0	41.3	41.5	41.8

Source: Jackson, A., and M. Pollock. "Practical Assessment of Body Composition." *The Physician and Sportsmedicine* (May 1985): 86. Reprinted with permission from McGraw-Hill, Inc.

Estimating Body Fat Percentages in Men: Sum of Chest, Abdomen, and Thigh Skinfolds

SUM OF SKINFOLDS (mm)	Age Groups								
	UNDER 22	23–27	28–32	33–37	38–42	43–47	48–52	53–57	OVER 58
8–10	1.3	1.8	2.3	2.9	3.4	3.9	4.5	5.0	5.5
11–13	2.2	2.8	3.3	3.9	4.4	4.9	5.5	6.0	6.5
14–16	3.2	3.8	4.3	4.8	5.4	5.9	6.4	7.0	7.5
17–19	4.2	4.7	5.3	5.8	6.3	6.9	7.4	8.0	8.5
20–22	5.1	5.7	6.2	6.8	7.3	7.9	8.4	8.9	9.5
23–25	6.1	6.6	7.2	7.7	8.3	8.8	9.4	9.9	10.5
26–28	7.0	7.6	8.1	8.7	9.2	9.8	10.3	10.9	11.4
29–31	8.0	8.5	9.1	9.6	10.2	10.7	11.3	11.8	12.4
32–34	8.9	9.4	10.0	10.5	11.1	11.6	12.2	12.8	13.3
35–37	9.8	10.4	10.9	11.5	12.0	12.6	13.1	13.7	14.3
38–40	10.7	11.3	11.8	12.4	12.9	13.5	14.1	14.6	15.2
41–43	11.6	12.2	12.7	13.3	13.8	14.4	15.0	15.5	16.1
44–46	12.5	13.1	13.6	14.2	14.7	15.3	15.9	16.4	17.0
47–49	13.4	13.9	14.5	15.1	15.6	16.2	16.8	17.3	17.9
50–52	14.3	14.8	15.4	15.9	16.5	17.1	17.6	18.2	18.8
53–55	15.1	15.7	16.2	16.8	17.4	17.9	18.5	19.1	19.7
56–58	16.0	16.5	17.1	17.7	18.2	18.8	19.4	20.0	20.5
59–61	16.9	17.4	17.9	18.5	19.1	19.7	20.2	20.8	21.4
62–64	17.6	18.2	18.8	19.4	19.9	20.5	21.1	21.7	22.2
65–67	18.5	19.0	19.6	20.2	20.8	21.3	21.9	22.5	23.1
68–70	19.3	19.9	20.4	21.0	21.6	22.2	22.7	23.3	23.9
71–73	20.1	20.7	21.2	21.8	22.4	23.0	23.6	24.1	24.7
74–76	20.9	21.5	22.0	22.6	23.2	23.8	24.4	25.0	25.5
77–79	21.7	22.2	22.8	23.4	24.0	24.6	25.2	25.8	26.3
80–82	22.4	23.0	23.6	24.2	24.8	25.4	25.9	26.5	27.1
83–85	23.2	23.8	24.4	25.0	25.5	26.1	26.7	27.3	27.9
86–88	24.0	24.5	25.1	25.7	26.3	26.9	27.5	28.1	28.7
89–91	24.7	25.3	25.9	26.5	27.1	27.6	28.2	28.8	29.4
92–94	25.4	26.0	26.6	27.2	27.8	28.4	29.0	29.6	30.2
95–97	26.1	26.7	27.3	27.9	28.5	29.1	29.7	30.3	30.9
98–100	26.9	27.4	28.0	28.6	29.2	29.8	30.4	31.0	31.6
101–103	27.5	28.1	28.7	29.3	29.9	30.5	31.1	31.7	32.3
104–106	28.2	28.8	29.4	30.0	30.6	31.2	31.8	32.4	33.0
107–109	28.9	29.5	30.1	30.7	31.3	31.9	32.5	33.1	33.7
110–112	29.6	30.2	30.8	31.4	32.0	32.6	33.2	33.8	34.4
113–115	30.2	30.8	31.4	32.0	32.6	33.2	33.8	34.5	35.1
116–118	30.9	31.5	32.1	32.7	33.3	33.9	34.5	35.1	35.7
119–121	31.5	32.1	32.7	33.3	33.9	34.5	35.1	35.7	36.4
122–124	32.1	32.7	33.3	33.9	34.5	35.1	35.8	36.4	37.0
125–127	32.7	33.3	33.9	34.5	35.1	35.8	36.4	37.0	37.6

Source: Pollock, M. L., D. H. Schmidt, and A. S. Jackson. "Measurement of Cardiorespiratory Fitness and Body Composition in the Clinical Setting." *Comprehensive Therapy* 6(9):12–27, 1980. Published with permission of the Laux Company, Inc., Harvard, Mass.

The Body Composition Analyzer

The body composition analyzer sends a mild electric impulse throughout the body and measures body density, determining the percentages of fat and lean body mass. A computer program is used to combine the electrical measurements with the input of a person's data, including age, gender, height, and weight. Standard equations are preprogrammed into the computer software to print out an estimate of the subject's percentage of body fat. Although this method is relatively new, the reliability and objectivity of this method seem to be good. However, like underwater weighing, this test can be expensive.

SOMATOTYPING

Somatotyping is the physical classification of the body. It determines the shape of your body and is something that cannot be changed, no matter how much you exercise or diet. Individuals can lose weight and change the shape of their muscles, but depending on their somatotype, they may still not attain their ideal physique. Generally, there are 3 descriptive body types: endomorph, mesomorph, and ectomorph (24).

Endomorph

The *endomorph* body type is characterized by a roundness and softness of the body, with small body contours and minimal definition of muscle tone. This is generally considered the "fatness" component of the body.

Mesomorph

The *mesomorph* body type is characterized by prominent musculature and a square body shape. The bones are large and covered with thick musculature. This is generally considered the "muscular" component of the body.

Ectomorph

The *ectomorph* body type is characterized predominantly by a linear body, which may look delicate or fragile. Bones are small, and the muscles are thin, not bulging. The arms and legs are relatively long compared to the trunk of the body. This is generally considered the "thinness" component of the body.

In Conclusion

Although body types are generally characterized into these three types, a single pure type does not really exist. Each of us is made up in part of all these three components, with different percentages of each. The dominant type that prevails is usually how we visualize our bodies.

With respect to body composition, the body can be changed in body fat content through aerobic exercise, toning, and diet. Unfortunately, we cannot change our body type, no matter how hard we try. You can rid yourself of any obsession to look thin by understanding these body composition principles. You can also stop using the scale to determine how fat you are. Leanness is what counts, *not* lightness.

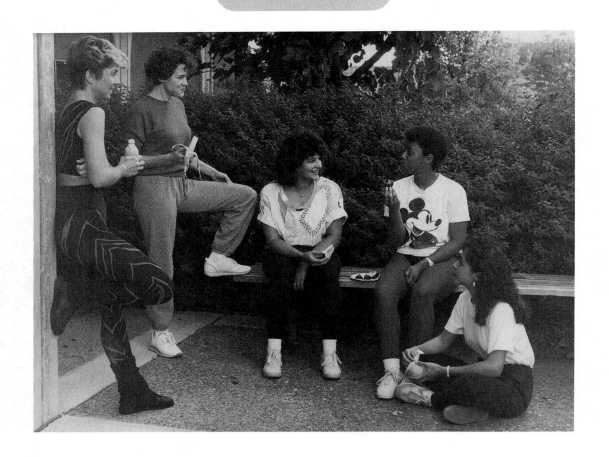

Nutrition
and Diet

Chapter

15

Nutrition is as important as exercise for staying in good health. The body cannot supply the strength and endurance needed for aerobic dance if it is not properly fueled. Rather than thinking in terms of "diet," which provokes a negative response from most people, you should develop good nutritional habits that you can maintain throughout the rest of your life. The old rule of eating a balanced selection of foods from the four basic food groups still applies.

A nutritionally adequate diet consists of:

1. Milk and milk products
2. Meats, fish, poultry, eggs, and substitutes of nuts and tofu and other soybean products
3. Fruits and vegetables
4. Breads and cereals

To fully understand the basics of proper nutrition, you should also become familiar with the types of nutrients that the body requires and their functions.

PROTEIN

The main function of protein is to build and repair body tissue; protein is the basic structural substance of each cell in the body. Protein is found in both animal and plant food sources. The animal food sources are meat, fish, poultry, eggs, milk, and milk products. The protein in animal food sources is called *complete* because it contains the eight amino acids essential to a well-balanced diet. These essential amino acids cannot be manufactured in the body and therefore must be supplied through the foods we eat. The plant food sources are lentils, legumes, nuts, cereals, and tofu and other soybean products. This *incomplete* protein lacks one or more of the essential amino acids. Most individual plant foods cannot supply the necessary total protein source; however, when properly combined, they can provide the essential amino acids, such as a combination of rice (grain) with beans (47).

Protein intake should comprise approximately 12 percent of daily total calories. This means 1 to 2 ounces of protein per day, or 0.9 grams of protein per kilogram of body weight (multiply your body weight in pounds by 0.424 to obtain your weight in kilograms) (44). Pregnant and nursing mothers are exceptions to this protein requirement; they should increase their protein intake by 10 and 20 grams, respectively (38).

When the intake of protein is excessive, the process of *deamination*—the breakdown of amino acids to fat—can be very stressful to the body. During deamination, nitrogen is released from the amino acids and quickly converted to ammonia. Ammonia is very toxic to the body and is therefore converted to urea, which is also toxic to the body, but to a lesser extent. For the body to eliminate urea, the urea must be diluted to urine. When the amount of urea is excessive, the body needs enormous amounts of water to dilute it to urine, so much so that even drinking endless glasses of water is not enough. To dilute the urea, the body gets the necessary water from its tissues. The end result is a stressful burden on the kidneys as they overwork to rid the body of urine (45).

Many Americans eat an excess of protein, primarily animal protein. Although animal protein in the diet is a good way of ensuring a balanced supply of essential amino acids, this protein is high in saturated fat (fats that are solid at room temperature) and cholesterol and not as easily digested as other forms of protein. Most nutritionists recommend reducing the consumption of animal protein and increasing the intake of plant (vegetable) protein.

FATS

Fats have the highest energy content of all nutrients. Fat's main function is to supply fuel and energy to the body, both at rest and during exercise. Fat has other functions as well: It cushions the body's vital organs, protects the body from extreme temperatures of cold, and helps in the utilization of the fat-soluble vitamins A, D, E, and K (47). Sources of fats include dairy products, meats, margarine, mayonnaise, nuts, seeds, and oils. However, two-thirds of fat intake should consist of nonsaturated and polyunsaturated fats, which are found in vegetables and such vegetable oils as corn, cottonseed, safflower, sesame seed, soybean, and sunflower seed.

Although there is no specific requirement for fat in the diet, there is a need for an essential fatty acid and the vitamins that are the components of fat. Currently, about 40 percent of Americans' daily caloric intake is composed of fat. A recommended dietary goal is less than 30 percent, with the amount of saturated fat in the diet less than 10 percent (49).

CARBOHYDRATES

Carbohydrates supply the body with its primary source of energy, glucose. Glucose (blood sugar) is the product of the digestion of carbohydrates and is stored in the muscles. Carbohydrates also provide fuel for the central nervous system and are a metabolic primer for fat metabolism (38).

Although all carbohydrates have a certain chemistry in common, there is a great deal of difference between one carbohydrate and another. The two general types of carbohydrates are simple and complex. *Simple carbohydrates*—sugars—are maltose, which is found in malt; lactose, found in milk; and sucrose, which is table sugar. When these sugars are ingested, they are converted to blood glucose almost immediately. Therefore, the consumption of simple carbohydrates causes blood glucose levels to fluctuate too quickly, making energy levels vacillate. Table sugar and the refined and processed sugars found in sodas, candy, cookies, cakes, and a realm of other sweetened treats offer no nutrients, are high in calories, and are associated with tooth decay, obesity, malnutrition, diabetes, and hypoglycemia (low blood sugar).

Complex carbohydrates—starches—are the natural sugars found in fruits, vegetables, and grains.

They are the best source of energy because they convert blood glucose slowly. In other words, they supply a sustained energy output.

Complex carbohydrates are probably the best foods we can eat because they are high in vitamins, minerals, and fiber. Fiber is the structural part of fruits, vegetables, legumes, cereals, and grains that humans cannot break down in the digestive system. It provides the roughage and bulk to keep the gastrointestinal tract working properly. Fiber has been shown to lower cholesterol and help control diabetes, and it may also help prevent colon cancer.

Daily caloric intake should include about 60 percent carbohydrates, with about half of that intake being complex carbohydrates. You should make every effort to decrease your intake of simple, "sugary" carbohydrates, which have no nutritional value, and increase your intake of complex carbohydrates, which offer vitamins, minerals, and fiber.

WATER

Water is second to oxygen as a substance necessary to sustain life. An adequate supply of water is necessary for all energy production in the body, for temperature control (especially during vigorous exercise), and for the elimination of waste products. *Dehydration,* or the loss of water in the body, can increase the risk of heat exhaustion and heatstroke (see the chart on page 146). You should include water as an essential part of your diet and be sure to drink water especially before and after exercise. When your teacher calls for a break during class, take the opportunity to get a drink from the water fountain or your water bottle. It is important to drink small amounts of water (½ to 1 cup) every 20 to 30 minutes during exercise. Drinking six to eight glasses of water a day is recommended for health maintenance. If you are physically active, you may need to drink more than eight glasses.

VITAMINS AND MINERALS

Vitamins help utilize and absorb other nutrients and are necessary for the body's normal metabolic functioning. Vitamins are classified as fat soluble or water soluble. *Fat-soluble vitamins* (A, D, E, and K) tend to remain stored in the body and are usually not excreted in the urine. An excess accumulation of these vitamins may be toxic to the body. *Water-soluble vitamins* (C and B complex) are excreted in the urine and are not stored in the body in appreciable amounts.

Minerals are the building materials for tissue and serve as body regulators. Two vitally important minerals are calcium and iron. Calcium is used to build bones and teeth. Iron is crucial in the formation of hemoglobin, the oxygen-carrying pigment in red blood cells. Both minerals are especially important to women: calcium as a preventer of osteoporosis and iron as a means to protect the body from iron-deficiency anemia. Vitamins and minerals are found in all food groups, especially in unrefined, unprocessed foods.

CALORIES

To maintain life and perform work, the body must have energy; the source of this energy is food. The energy food releases is measured in *calories,* or more specifically, **kilocalories.** The number of calories the body needs varies widely among individuals.

Virtually all the calories of energy the body uses are supplied by carbohydrates, fats, and proteins. Carbohydrates are the body's primary energy source. Fats, second to carbohydrates as a fuel source, are utilized if the carbohydrate supply is too low to meet the body's basic energy needs. Proteins provide an alternate energy source; the body uses them only when there are not enough calories available in the form of carbohydrates and fats. Protein is rarely used as an energy source; its most important function is to aid the body's growth and repair.

The amount of calories the body requires depends on the amount of calories (energy) it expends. You gain weight if you consume more calories in food than you use during activity. You lose weight if your caloric intake is less than the number of calories your body uses during activity. How much energy (the number of calories) you need in a day depends on your age, size, and activity level.

Adverse Effects of Dehydration

Percentage of
Body Weight Loss

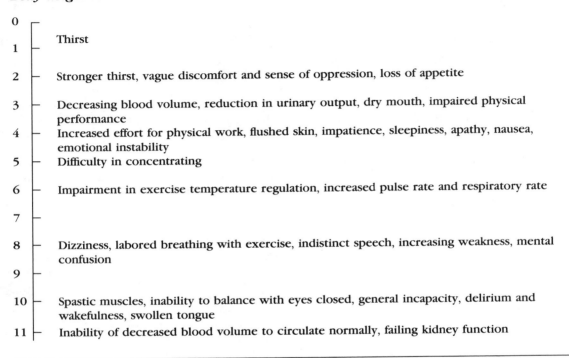

0	
1	Thirst
2	Stronger thirst, vague discomfort and sense of oppression, loss of appetite
3	Decreasing blood volume, reduction in urinary output, dry mouth, impaired physical performance
4	Increased effort for physical work, flushed skin, impatience, sleepiness, apathy, nausea, emotional instability
5	Difficulty in concentrating
6	Impairment in exercise temperature regulation, increased pulse rate and respiratory rate
7	
8	Dizziness, labored breathing with exercise, indistinct speech, increasing weakness, mental confusion
9	
10	Spastic muscles, inability to balance with eyes closed, general incapacity, delirium and wakefulness, swollen tongue
11	Inability of decreased blood volume to circulate normally, failing kidney function

Reference: Greenleaf, J. E. "The Body's Need for Fluids." In *Nutrition and Athletic Performance: Proceedings of the Conference on Nutritional Determinants in Athletic Performance,* edited by W. Haskell, J. Scala, and J. Whittam. Palo Alto, CA: Bull Publishing Company, 1982. *Source: Nutrition for Living.* Menlo Park, CA: Addison-Wesley, 1985, p. 76.

It is also true that not all nutrients are of equal caloric value. One food of equal weight to another can contain more calories just because of its value. A caloric value chart follows:

Nutrient	Caloric Value
Protein	4 calories per gram
Carbohydrate	4 calories per gram
Fat	9 calories per gram
Alcohol	7 calories per gram

It is obvious that fat is the most calorically expensive nutrient; therefore, the amount of fat in the diet should be limited.

As mentioned earlier, in a balanced diet, 10 to 15 percent of the calories should be protein; 50 to 60 percent, carbohydrate; and 30 percent, fat. As you become involved in aerobic dance, you should intelligently evaluate your body's calorie needs and balance those needs with correct nutritional requirements. To evaluate your diet, keep an accurate record of foods eaten and the number of calories in each food. Your record should show the total amount of calories consumed, with separate categories indicating how many calories were protein, carbohydrate, and fat.

An example of how to determine the caloric value of food items is outlined below.

A piece of whole wheat bread that contains 2 grams of fat, 13 grams of carbohydrate, and 3 grams of protein would supply the following number of calories:

2 grams of fat = 18 calories
13 grams of carbohydrate = 52 calories
3 grams of protein = 12 calories
Caloric total = 80 calories
Approximately 23 percent fat
Approximately 64 percent carbohydrate
Approximately 13 percent protein

If your record shows an imbalance among categories, make a change in your eating habits (27).

In addition to maintaining a balanced diet, you must have a balance between your total food intake and your exercise output. If your total food intake and exercise output are consistently balanced, you will maintain your weight.

If you want to gain or lose weight, either increase or decrease your total food intake while maintaining your output of exercise. In other words, to lose weight, you must consume fewer calories; to gain weight, you must consume more calories. The best way to lose weight is to combine changed eating habits with a good aerobic exercise program.

A pound of stored fat equals 3,500 calories. Thus, to lose 1 pound per week, you must decrease your daily caloric intake by 500 calories; to lose 2 pounds per week, you must decrease your daily intake by 1,000 calories:

1-lb fat loss per week = 3,500 calories eliminated from diet
= 3,500 calories ÷ 7 days
= 500 calories/day eliminated from diet

2-lb fat loss per week = 7,000 calories eliminated from diet
= 7,000 calories ÷ 7 days
= 1,000 calories/day eliminated from diet

Weight loss should involve a weight-reduction program that is consistent and evenly paced.

WEIGHT LOSS, OR THE "SET POINT" THEORY

If weight loss were merely a reflection of decreasing total caloric intake by diet, it would certainly be a simple matter to lose weight. Although weight loss normally occurs at the onset of a diet, the body's weight tends to stabilize at some new, lower level. To continue to lose weight becomes difficult. Long-term weight control is explained by new insights of weight control in the "set point" theory.

The set point theory maintains that the brain's hypothalamus regulates weight by comparing the body's current level of fat with a kind of constant internal standard. When a person's fat level falls below this internal standard, the body responds with increased appetite. If food intake is not increased, the body adjusts its metabolic rate to protect its usual level of fat stores. During a diet, when food intake is not increased to meet the body's increased appetite demands, the body adjusts its metabolic rate by burning calories more slowly. When a dieter resumes normal eating patterns, it is not uncommon to experience weight regain due to the body's slower metabolic rate.

The body's slower metabolic rate also affects the total fat-burning capacity of the body. The slowdown of the body's fat-burning capacity is due partly to a decrease in lean body mass, or muscle. During dieting, much of the weight loss occurs from the fat that is burned in muscle tissue. Finally, dieting causes enzyme changes in the adipose tissue lipoprotein lipase (a fat-storing enzyme). When caloric intake is decreased, this enzyme is dramatically increased, causing the body to become more efficient at storing fat.

Rather than attempting to lose weight through dieting, the set point theory maintains that to lose weight, the body's set point must be lowered. The most effective way to lower the set point is through exercise. Once the set point is lowered, the body will work to maintain the lower fat level, just as it tried to maintain the higher fat level described in the dieting process. As opposed to dieting, weight loss through exercise maintains muscle mass. Remember that most fat is burned within the muscle. Through exercise, fat is lost; thus the ratio of muscle to fat is increased. The increased ratio of muscle to fat also has long-term benefits since muscle requires more calories than fat to maintain itself.

Exercise also changes the enzymes of the muscle system to be more effective in burning fat. Oxidative enzymes are increased as a result of moderate aerobic exercise, thus increasing the ability of the muscles to burn fat and to lose fat stores.

With respect to the set point theory, the type of exercise for weight control is crucial. Aerobic exercise is the most beneficial because it allows the body to burn fat effectively during exercise. For weight loss, aerobic exercise must be done at a moderate pace and at least five days a week. Although research indicates that three days a week yields an aerobic effect, four days a week appears to be the threshold for weight loss, while six to seven days a week seems to be the ideal.

WEIGHT LOSS FALLACIES

Weight loss programs are promoted by every avenue of media possible. Promises of simple and easy methods of weight loss and body toning are weekly features. Avoid fad diets, many of which can produce hazardous health problems. Never eliminate calories totally from one food group, as is called for in many fad diets. If you lose weight quickly, your body does not have enough time to adapt to the lower calorie intake, so you usually gain back the lost weight. And diets that promote quick weight loss by the elimination of water cause dehydration and the loss of important minerals (30).

Other beauty claims of weight loss include spot reduction, or the removal of fat from one area. Fat can only be eliminated proportionally as a result of overall weight loss. For most women, by virtue of heredity or female hormones, the thighs and abdomen carry a protective layer of fat. These areas seem to be the first where fat appears and the last for fat to disappear during any change in body weight. Claims to eliminate fat from one specific area are yet another weight loss fallacy.

A nutritionally balanced diet will best help the body respond to the physical demands placed on it during aerobic dance. The following sample menus, not "diets," are based on sound nutritional concepts.

Menu 1

Meal	Calories	Meal	Calories
BREAKFAST		**DINNER**	
2 slices whole wheat toast	120	6 oz chicken, white meat, no skin	290
1 poached egg	80	1 medium baked potato	90
1 oz cream cheese	105	1 pat butter	50
6 oz orange juice	90	lettuce salad	30
coffee or tea with 1 oz lowfat milk	20	1 T blue cheese dressing	90
	415	1 C steamed broccoli	60
		1 C peach slices	65
		with ½ C lowfat yogurt	75
			750
LUNCH			
hamburger pattie 4 oz	250	**SNACK**	
½ C creamed cottage cheese	120	3 C plain popcorn	165
1 rye roll	60	*or*	
celery sticks	15	1 oz cheddar cheese	100
1 medium apple	80	with 4 Triscuit crackers	88
	525		188

Total calories for the day   1,855 or 1,878

Menu 2

Meal	Calories	Meal	Calories
BREAKFAST		**DINNER**	
½ C oatmeal	150	8 oz perch, meat only	260
½ C lowfat milk	65	1 T tartar sauce	75
½ grapefruit	60	1 C cooked brown rice	200
1 slice whole wheat toast	60	8 spears steamed asparagus	30
1 pat butter	50	1 C strawberries	60
coffee or tea with 1 oz lowfat milk	20	with 1 T light cream	50
	405		675
LUNCH		**SNACK**	
turkey sandwich:		1 C plain lowfat yogurt	130
2 slices whole wheat bread	120	with 1 T wheatgerm,	100
4 oz turkey	230	½ C applesauce, unsweetened	50
1 oz mayonnaise	100		280
lettuce	10		
1 banana	100		
carrot sticks	20		
	580	Total calories for the day	1,940

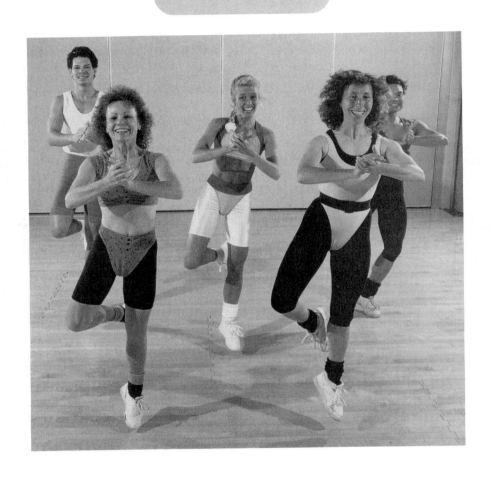

Adding Variety to Your Aerobic Workout

Chapter

16

In this chapter we will describe three ways you can add variety to your workout. These methods can be added to your regular routine and will keep you motivated for a long time!

STEP WORKOUT

The **step workout** is a type of aerobic conditioning class that uses a low bench as its cornerstone. Bench heights can range from 4 to 14 inches. Benches should be sturdy as well as slip- and skid-proof. You can make your own bench or purchase one of the commercial brands that are available through catalogs or fitness supply stores. An adjustable bench is recommended because, as you improve, the bench can be raised for a more demanding workout.

The step provides a low-impact, high-energy workout that puts added emphasis on your calves, thighs, and buttocks. In this workout, you perform a series of routines in which you step up and down from the bench in time to the music. As your fitness level improves, you can adjust the height of the bench, increase the tempo of the music, and use hand-held weights.

In a typical class, the warm-up will usually begin without the bench. The bench, though, can double as a warm-up/cool-down prop, on which you can sit, lie, or lean for stretching or calisthenics. Once your body is warmed and stretched, you can begin the step workout.

The basic step is right foot up, left foot up, right foot down, left foot down. Once this basic movement is rhythmically and physically comfortable, you can add variations. Your instructor might lead you up and over the other side of the bench, up with a knee lift or a kick, and eventually up and into a hop or small jump. The combinations can be as varied as in a typical aerobics class. You can approach the bench from any of its sides, vary the movement of the free leg, experiment with rhythmical patterns, and alternate arm patterns.

A step class is not recommended for the beginner. A reasonable level of fitness is encouraged since stepping is more intense than walking or even running on flat ground.

Certain step techniques are encouraged to prevent injury:

1. Make sure you place your whole foot on the step.
2. Bend your knees at all times when stepping.
3. Keep the step in your line of vision at all times.
4. Warm up thoroughly before beginning the aerobic phase. Especially concentrate on your calves, quadriceps, hamstrings, buttock muscles, and lower back.
5. Do not perform a step workout as your first exercise experience—become an experienced exerciser, and then do the step!
6. Individuals with knee problems are not encouraged to do the step because it places stress on the knees. Consult your doctor before you participate.

The step workout appeals to both men and women; it adds variety to their fitness programs, provides a total body workout, and is vigorous enough for a maximum challenge.

INTERVAL TRAINING

Interval training is a method of conditioning that has been used to train athletes for many years. Recently it has been implemented in aerobic dance classes as an alternative to the usual routine, as a way to increase exercise intensity and hence aerobic capacity.

Interval training is a series of high-intensity exercises alternated with periods of light or mild exercise. This method of training allows the body to adjust to the more intense work load by alternating it with lighter exercise, and at the same time it improves conditioning by making greater than normal demands on the body.

The important terms that define an interval training program are listed below:

Work interval—this is the high-intensity work load portion of the workout. The body works at the high end of its target heart range. It should last no more than 90 seconds.

Rest interval—this segment follows the work interval. During this phase, the body works at the lowest end of its target heart range. The rest interval usually lasts twice as long as the work interval. The timing of this interval depends on the intensity of the work interval. The more intense work load will require a longer rest interval.

Sets—these are a series of work and rest intervals. One set might be a 90-second work interval followed by a 3-minute rest interval, performed 3 times.

Repetitions—these are the number of work-rest intervals within one set. Using the above example, there are 3 repetitions that constitute one set.

So how can interval training be used for aerobic dance? The aerobic phase of the class can be set up as an interval training program. It should begin with a rest interval serving as a warm-up period to progressively increase the heart rate, using low-impact moves such as walking, marching, and light jogging. The music should range from 130 to 140 BPM. The heart rate should be sustained at 60 to 70 percent of its maximum. The work interval should utilize big locomotor movements such as hops, jumps, and leaps. The music for this phase should range from 145 to 165 BPM, allowing the heart rate to achieve 80 to 90 percent of its maximum.

For a 27-minute aerobic workout, you could do a work interval of 90 seconds followed by a rest interval of 3 minutes, with six repetitions completing one set. You can vary the length of time for the work and rest intervals, but in order to work and improve the aerobic energy system, a ratio of 1:2 for the work-rest intervals is necessary.

Interval Training Programs for an Aerobic Dance Class

Work Interval	Rest Interval	Sets	Repetitions	Total Time
90 seconds	3 minutes	1	6	27 minutes
90 seconds	3 minutes	2	3	27 minutes
75 seconds	2½ minutes	1	8	30 minutes
75 seconds	2½ minutes	2	4	30 minutes
60 seconds	2 minutes	1	10	30 minutes
60 seconds	2 minutes	2	5	30 minutes

Interval training is not appropriate for the beginner. It is best suited to the aerobic dancer who needs to increase the intensity of his or her current workout or who wants variety in his or her present exercise regime.

The chart above defines interval programs for aerobic dance. You can also create your own program using the principles described.

CIRCUIT TRAINING

Circuit training is not new. However, aerobic circuit training has now become a widely popular class format for aerobic enthusiasts. **Circuit training** consists of a number of "stations," where a specific exercise or routine is performed in a given period of time. Once the exercise is completed, the participant moves quickly to the next station, also performed in a specific time frame. Once all the stations have been completed, the circuit is finished. Aerobic circuit training combines aerobic exercise (to build cardiorespiratory endurance) with weight-training exercises (to develop muscular strength and endurance). By alternating aerobic and weight-training exercise stations, this combined workout can provide maximum benefits.

It is important that the sequencing of exercises in a circuit be arranged so that no two consecutive stations work the same muscle group. By placing aerobic stations between the strength stations, you develop your cardiovascular endurance as well as your strength. However, to maintain the

elevated heart rate achieved at the aerobic stations, you must move quickly from one station to the next. It is also important that strength-training exercises be performed at an "aerobic" pace, using light weights and quick repetitions. The emphasis on weight-training work is to develop muscular endurance rather than power.

The format for an aerobic circuit training session is based on timed intervals at each station, which will be determined by your instructor. Each station usually takes 45 to 75 seconds. You attempt to do as many repetitions as you can within that time slot. After completing that station, you go to the next one directly, or when the instructor calls "change."

Another method for integrating an aerobic circuit program into an aerobics class is to perform 10 minutes of aerobics with the group and then complete a strength circuit for 10 minutes. Repeat this sequence for the length of the class. In both methods, be sure to warm up and cool down!

One of the many advantages of aerobic circuit training is the versatility of the program. Students may work with a class, individually, or in a buddy system—with another classmate or the instructor. Workout programs can be tailored to meet individual goals by making different stations of the workout more or less intense. In order to overload a circuit class you may:

1. Increase the number of stations
2. Increase the number of repetitions performed at each station by increasing the duration or pace

3. Repeat the number of times the circuit is repeated
4. Increase the amount of weight used

Two examples of a circuit workout are outlined below. One circuit consists entirely of strength stations, with a normal aerobic routine performed at the beginning, middle, or end of the circuit. The second circuit alternates between strength and aerobic stations. Use weights where it is applicable, and remember to go quickly from one station to the next. Do as many repetitions as the time will allow, but do not sacrifice technique for speed!

		Circuit One (Conditioning)	*Circuit Two (Aerobics with Conditioning)*
STATION	1	Squat with upright row	Jumping jacks
STATION	2	Push-up	Squat with lateral raise
STATION	3	Lunge with bicep curl	Jog in place
STATION	4	Abdominal curl	Lunge with bicep curl
STATION	5	Bent leg lift	Alternating knee lift and kick
STATION	6	Forward arm raise	Abdominal curl
STATION	7	Tricep kickback	Jump-roping in place
STATION	8	Side thigh lift	Push-up
STATION	9	Abdominal curl	Clap over and under leg
STATION	10	Inner thigh lift	Side thigh lift
STATION	11	Heel raise with side lateral raise	Bench-stepping

APPENDIX A
Frequently Asked Questions and the Answers You Want to Hear

QUESTION 1

If during exercise your heart rate is above your target zone and you feel good, how is this harmful? Should you pace down to your target zone?

This question about working *above* your "target zone" is a very important one. To answer it, we must consider this fact: The heart is a muscle.

When you begin aerobic dance, you see the teacher and other students working effortlessly at a rapid pace; you are distracted by the rhythmic music that carries you forward into movement; and you come into the class with a firm commitment to "just do it!" You can very easily find your heart beating way above your target zone, and yet you are "feeling no pain." This is, in fact, a dangerous physical state to remain in for any length of time. Your heart, like any other muscle, can sustain just so many repetitions before fatigue and muscle collapse occur. This is one of the reasons why your aerobic instructor reminds you throughout the class to stay in your *safe* target or training zone (65 to 85 percent of your maximum heart rate).

On the other hand, it is important to understand that heart rate is not the only way to measure intensity, and sometimes it is misleading and inappropriate for the individual. Some people can achieve high heart rates without working too hard; this is normal for them. If this is the case, then using the talk test and perceived exertion would be more accurate ways to measure the intensity of your workout. If your heart rate is continually high and you do feel good, perhaps it would be wise to check with a physician to see if this high pulse is normal for you.

QUESTION 2

If working at the target heart rate is good training, wouldn't working over the target rate be better? Can you eventually adjust to a higher target heart rate?

Working above your target heart rate would not be appropriate for aerobic exercise because this intensity of exercise would be too difficult to maintain for any period of time. If you only have 20 minutes to workout, or if you are involved in competitive training, increasing your intensity to the high end of your target range would be beneficial. If you are exercising to burn fat, you want to work for a longer duration and a moderate intensity. Working faster, however, is not beneficial for improving your cardiorespiratory endurance; you want to increase your duration but stay within the target zone.

You can adjust to a higher target zone as you get more fit, because your body will have to work harder to get the same results you achieved when you were less fit. You will also find that your heart rate will be slower and you will feel less and less fatigued over a longer distance because your heart muscle is stronger.

QUESTION 3

What is the importance of a warm-up in aerobic activity?

Before beginning any exercise program, it is important to allow time for the body to shift from a resting state to a moving, active state. Usually the most effective warm-up is one that gradually works into the exercise program.

The warm-up should result in an increase of heart rate as well as an increase in the temperature of the muscles. Also, a proper warm-up before peak activity reduces the chances of muscle injury and soreness.

QUESTION 4

Will jogging produce the same cardiovascular and weight loss effect as high-impact aerobics?

Yes, jogging and high-impact aerobics have the same effect on cardiovascular efficiency and weight loss. All aerobic exercises deal with the heart and lungs. As long as an exercise is vigorous enough to sustain the heart rate in your target zone for the suggested 20-minute (minimum) time period and you exercise at least 3 days per week, you will notice beneficial changes in cardiovascular efficiency. With regard to weight loss, remember that calorie intake has to be balanced against calorie output; you will have to monitor what you eat as well as how many calories you burn with exercise. However, proper nutrition cannot be maintained in diets of fewer than 1,200 kilocalories per day. To lose weight successfully, start with a nutritious diet, and then balance it

with enough exercise to use more calories than you eat.

Compare the following activities performed by a person weighing 130 lb:

Dancing (choreographed, vigorous)	9.9 kilocalories per minute
Running (cross-country)	9.6 kilocalories per minute
Running (in place)	21.0 kilocalories per minute

The more a person weighs, the more kilocalories are burned per minute; also, the more vigorous or faster the activity, the more kilocalories are burned per minute. Remember that for weight loss to occur, aerobic exercise should be performed 5 to 7 days a week. This will supply the appropriate output for weight loss and will change the metabolic rate.

QUESTION 5

If you feel pain from a previous injury, should you stop exercising or "work through it"?

Pain is a good indication that something is wrong. If you are recovering from an injury, you should carefully monitor the intensity of the exercise during the rehabilitation period. Although slight discomfort may be felt as you renew an exercise program after recuperating from an injury, you should not feel pain per se. If this does occur, stop and give your body more time to heal.

QUESTION 6

Can body toning be of any benefit to someone who is overweight? Can you tone muscles that you can't even see?

First of all, body toning will not rid the body of fat. Only aerobic exercise will burn fat. Body toning merely tones up the muscles under the fat. The exercises performed in the body toning section of class are important as they contour and tone the muscles, giving the figure shape and form. Strong muscles also help to achieve good posture, which can improve the image of the body. Muscles that are not used regularly will atrophy, giving the figure a loose or flabby look. Even though the muscles are hidden, regular body toning sessions are important for improving muscular strength and the look of your figure.

QUESTION 7

Should I exercise when I have my period?

As a general rule, there is no problem with exercising during menstruation. In fact, it can help to get the circulation moving and can actually make you feel more energetic. In some cases though, with heavy cramping, if it is very uncomfortable to move, rest would be encouraged. In this case, it is advisable to see a physician to help you through the pain.

QUESTION 8

Should I exercise when I have a cold?

This, of course, is a very individual situation. Sometimes with a slight cold, exercise may help to relieve some of the aches and pains and make you feel better. A severe cold, on the other hand, would leave you without the adequate strength and energy required for a workout. If indeed you do decide to exercise, remember to check your heart rate, and exercise at a moderate workout level. Also, fluids are extremely important. Be sure to drink plenty of water throughout the workout. Juices high in vitamin C are good to drink before or after the workout.

If you are uncomfortable during the workout, *stop*. Resume your workout program when you are in better health.

QUESTION 9

What is a good snack to eat before an aerobic workout? How soon before the class should I eat?

A preexercise snack should consist mainly of complex carbohydrates, such as breads, grains, pastas, fruits, and vegetables, since these foods are easily digested. High-carbohydrate foods provide quick energy to the muscles and also quickly replenish energy stores after exercise. Avoid high-sugar foods, such as soft drinks, candy, and other sweets. Soon after these foods are eaten, when the "sugar high" stops, your blood sugar level will dramatically drop, leaving you feeling tired and sluggish. Although individuals differ, generally it is recommended to have a snack not less than 1 to 2 hours before a workout.

QUESTION 10

Can I continue with my aerobic dance workouts while I am pregnant?

There is no reason not to continue exercising while you are pregnant, as long as you listen to your body, exercise moderately, and are under the regular care of a physician. Exercise that raises the heart rate to 140 beats per minute is generally considered moderate. Exercise at the higher end of the target zone entails some risk. The American College of Obstetricians and Gynecologists has set forth guidelines for exercising safely during pregnancy. Basically, the guidelines suggest the following:

Be sure to warm up before and cool down after all exercise.
Monitor your heart rate or use the perceived exertion test during all phases of the workout. Your physician should establish target zones, which should not be exceeded.
Exercise regularly; a program of at least 3 times a week is preferable to intermittent activity.
Avoid ballistic movements.
Avoid deep flexion and extension of the joints due to connective tissue laxity.
Drink liquids throughout your exercise workout to prevent dehydration.
If any unusual symptoms occur, stop all activity and consult your physician (2).

For more explicit details pertaining to your individual situation, consult your physician.

QUESTION 11

Why do I sweat? Why do I sweat more when I have stopped exercising?

Sweating is your body's way of cooling you off. When your muscles contract, 25 percent of the energy produced is for movement, whereas the other 75 percent is converted to heat. If your body were not able to reduce this heat through sweat, serious consequences could develop.

During exercise, more blood is needed at the muscles, so it is shunted from the skin; this causes a build-up of heat. When we stop exercising, the body can send additional blood to the skin. We perspire more profusely then to dissipate the excess heat produced. In addition, while we are participating in vigorous exercise, our sweat evaporates, which increases the efficiency of our cooling mechanism.

QUESTION 12

What is the correct way to breath during exercise?

The important thing to remember is to breath naturally and to allow the breath to come in and leave through both your nose and mouth at a rate that feels comfortable. Never hold your breath when you exercise since this can cause dizziness and fainting. The demands of the exercise will determine the rate and depth of the breath. During conditioning exercises, though, it is important to exhale on the exertion.

QUESTION 13

Why do I sometimes get a side pain when I exercise, and what should I do when this occurs?

The answer to this question is not totally understood. One theory states that the pain is caused by trapped metabolic gases that create pressure in this area and therefore pain. The other theory states that there is a lack of oxygen reaching the respiratory muscles, thereby causing a cramp in the diaphragm area. Whatever the case, the best way to deal with this pain, or "side stitch," is to

stop vigorous exercise and walk slowly until it subsides. As your fitness level improves, this situation will occur less frequently.

QUESTION 14

How does smoking affect my ability to exercise?

When you smoke, you inhale carbon monoxide. Hemoglobin, the protein molecule that carries oxygen to the muscles, has a stronger attachment to carbon monoxide than it does to oxygen; so if carbon monoxide is present in the lungs, the amount of oxygen carried by hemoglobin to the muscles will be reduced. Cigarette smoking also decreases the airflow in and out of the lungs. Both of these situations will make endurance-type exercise more difficult to sustain.

QUESTION 15

Should I exercise in the heat?

When you exercise in the heat, your body has a more difficult time dissipating the internal heat because the external environment does not supply any relief. Profuse sweating often results and with it, a large amount of water loss. This could result in dehydration and, more seriously, heat exhaustion or heat stroke. It is acceptable, though, to exercise in the heat; yet the following precautions must be taken:

Decrease the intensity of exercise beyond 30 minutes.
Exercise in the early morning or late evening.
Drink plenty of fluids before, during, and after exercising.
Wear lightweight and well-ventilated clothing to expose as much skin as possible to aid in the evaporation of sweat.

APPENDIX B
Sources for Fitness Evaluations

Fitness evaluation tests and charts are used at the teacher's discretion.

TESTS

A number of valid tests can be used to evaluate your level of fitness; we recommend the following references.

Endurance Tests

1.5 mile test: Cooper, Kenneth H. *The Aerobics Way*. New York: M. Evans, 1977.

3-minute step test: Y.M.C.A. of the U.S.A., *3-Minute Step Test*, 101 N. Wacker Drive, Chicago, IL 60606.

Strength Tests

Abdominal strength: Y.M.C.A. of the U.S.A., *Abdominal Strength Test*, 101 N. Wacker Drive, Chicago, IL 60606.

Arm strength: Krepton, Dorie, and Donald Chu. *Everybody's Aerobic Book*. Edina, MN: Bellwether Press, 1986.

Leg strength: Krepton, Dorie, and Donald Chu. *Everybody's Aerobic Book*. Edina, MN: Bellwether Press, 1986.

Flexibility

Shoulder lift: Bucher, Charles A., and William E. Prentice. *Fitness for College and Life*. St. Louis: Mosby, 1985.

Sit and reach: Bucher, Charles A., and William E. Prentice. *Fitness for College and Life*. St. Louis: Mosby, 1985.

Trunk extension: Hockey, R. V. *Physical Fitness*. 5th ed. St. Louis Times Mirror/Mosby, 1985.

Hip flexion and hamstring mobility: Krepton, Dorie, and Donald Chu. *Everybody's Aerobic Book*. Edina, MN: Bellwether Press, 1986.

Body Composition

Skinfold test: *Research Quarterly for Exercise and Sport* 52 (1981).

CHARTS

The following charts are of value to the teacher and student as a means of personal evaluation. Feel free to duplicate these forms.

Student Profile

N A M E _____

A D D R E S S _____

P H O N E _____

Rate your fitness level:

_____ Superior   _____ Fair

_____ Excellent   _____ Poor

_____ Good   _____ Very poor

Previous instruction in aerobic dance _____

Sports/exercise in which you participate _____

Reasons for taking this course _____

Did anyone recommend this course or instructor? _____

Your physical limitations _____

Activity or type of exercise you would like to have covered _____

_____

Your heart rate:

_____ Resting

_____ Target

Do you smoke? _____ If so, how many cigarettes per day? _____

List your favorite kind of music, favorite song, favorite singer or group _____

_____

List your interests _____

_____

Body Measurement

N A M E_____

Procedure: Measure each area at its widest part.

Measurements

Area	Initial	After 8 weeks	After 16 weeks
Weight			
Biceps	R L	R L	R L
Chest			
Waist			
Abdomen			
Hips			
Thighs	R L	R L	R L
Calves	R L	R L	R L
Ankles	R L	R L	R L

APPENDIX C
Music Resources

Any record store will have a wide variety of aerobic music. The choice is what appeals to you. Rhythmic and upbeat music is most appropriate for much of the class; however, the flexibility cool-down segment is best suited to slow, mellow music that encourages relaxation. Besides record stores, there are many companies nationwide that make audio tapes specifically for aerobic classes. Following is a list of companies that provide this service:

1. Aerobics Power Mix
   Power Productions, Inc.
   P.O. Box 3812
   Gaithersburg, MD 20878
   1-800-777-Beat
2. In-Lytes Productions
   P.O. Box 70125
   Louisville, KY 40270
   502-589-PUMP
3. David Shelton Productions
   P.O. Box 652
   Layton, UT 84041
   1-800-272-3411

4. Dancetracks!
   AE1 Music Network, Inc.
   72 Spring St., Suite 1004
   New York, NY 10012
   1-800-AE1-MUSIC
5. Muscle Mixes Aerobic Music Service
   2934 Northwood Blvd.
   Orlando, FL 32803
   1-800-52-Mixes
6. Pacesetter Music
   P.O. Box 57
   5472 S. 7100 W.
   Hooper, UT 84315-0057
   801-773-2000
7. Musicflex Inc.
   163-35 98th St.
   Queens, NY 11414
   718-738-MUFX
8. Mix Music International Inc.
   P.O. Box 2452
   Kankakee, IL 60901
   1-800-733-3049
9. Ken Alan Associates
   7985 Santa Monica Blvd., #109
   Los Angeles, CA 90046
   213-659-2503

APPENDIX D
Suggested Reading

AEROBICS AND FITNESS

Allsen, Phillip E., Joyce M. Harrison, and Barbara Vance. *Fitness for Life.* Dubuque, IA: Brown, 1983.

Bailey, Covert. *Fit or Fat.* Boston: Houghton Mifflin, 1978.

Cooper, Kenneth H. *Aerobics for Women.* New York: Bantam, 1980.

———. *The Aerobics Program for Total Well-Being.* New York: Bantam, 1983.

Cooper, Phyllis Gorney, ed. *Aerobics: Theory and Practice.* Costa Mesa, CA: HDL Publishing, 1988.

Donovan, Grant, Jane McNamara, and Peter Gianoli. *Exercise Danger.* Dubuque, IA: Kendall/Hunt, 1988.

Fox, Edward, Timothy Kirby, and Ann Roberts Fox. *Bases of Fitness.* New York: Macmillan, 1987.

Gelder, Naneene Van. *Aerobic Dance-Exercise Instructor Manual.* San Diego: IDEA Foundation, 1987.

Getchell, Bud. *Physical Fitness: A Way of Life.* New York: Wiley, 1983.

Greggains, Joanie. *Joanie Greggains' Total Shape Up.* New York: New American Library, 1984.

Kravitz, Len. *Anybody's Guide to Total Fitness.* Dubuque, IA: Kendall/Hunt, 1989.

McIntosh, Mathew. *Lifetime Aerobics.* Dubuque, IA: William C. Brown, 1990.

Miller, D., and E. Allen. *Fitness: A Lifetime Concept.* Minneapolis: Burgess, 1982.

Shape Magazine, Shape Magazine Inc., 21100 Erwin St., Woodland Hills, CA 91367

Smith, Kathy. *Ultimate Workout.* New York: Bantam, 1983.

Thaxton, Nolan. *Pathways to Fitness.* New York: Harper and Row, 1988.

FLEXIBILITY

Anderson, Bob. *Stretching.* Blinds, CA: Shelter Publications, 1980.

Benjamin, Ben E. *Sports Without Pain.* New York: Summit Books, 1979.

INJURIES

Arnheim, D. *Modern Principles of Athletic Training,* 7th ed. St. Louis: Times Mirror/Mosby, 1985.

Fahey, Tom. *Athletic Training: Principles and Practice.* Palo Alto, CA: Mayfield, 1986.

Morris, A. *Sports Medicine: Prevention of Athletic Injuries.* Dubuque, IA: Brown, 1984.

Ritter, M. A., and M. J. Albohm. *Your Injury: A Commonsense Guide to the Management of Sports Injury.* Indianapolis: Benchmark, 1987.

Solomon, Ruth, Sandra Minton, and John Solomon. *Preventing Dance Injuries.* Waldorf, MD: American Alliance, 1990.

Wright, S. *Dancer's Guide to Injuries of the Lower Extremities.* New York: Cornwall Books, 1985.

NUTRITION

Bailey, Covert. *Fit or Fit Target Diet.* Boston: Houghton Mifflin, 1984.

Brody, Jane. *Jane Brody's Nutrition Book.* New York: Bantam, 1981.

———. *Jane Brody's Good Food Book: Living the High Carbohydrate Way.* New York: W. W. Norton, 1985.

Clark, Nancy. *The Athlete's Kitchen.* New York: Bantam, 1983.

———. *Sports Nutrition Guidebook.* Chicago: Leisure, 1990.

Dusky, Lorraine, and J. J. Leedy. *How to Eat Like a Thin Person.* New York: Simon and Schuster, 1982.

Franz, M. J. *Fast Food Facts.* Minneapolis: International Diabetes Center, 1987.

Tribole, Evelyn. *Eating on the Run.* Champaign, IL: Life Enhancement, 1987.

Whitney, Eleanor Noss, and Eva May Hamilton. *Nutrition: Concepts and Controversies.* St. Paul: West, 1982.

APPENDIX E
Video Cassette Workouts

If you are building a fitness library or merely want to rent a video for a home workout, you will want to select a video that includes a well-rounded workout program, with sound instructional techniques and safety standards. Consider the following criteria for evaluating a video:

Does the workout include an adequate warm-up and cool-down stretch?

Is the workout appropriate for your participation level, or are there a variety of levels to select from?

Does the instructor provide heart rate checks during the aerobic activity?

Does the instructor perform movements using proper technique?

Is there clear cueing for movements by the instructor?

Does the tape have good audiovisual quality with easy to follow camera angles?

Does the workout include exercises for opposing muscle groups?

Does the instructor include safety precautions for exercises?

Is the overall presentation and workout motivational?

The following selection of aerobic workout video cassettes is suggested. A short description of the video is provided to help you choose a workout that is appropriate for you. For a more complete list, you can send away for the catalog entitled *The Complete Guide to Exercise Videos* (College Video Specialities Inc., 5390 Main Street, NE, Dept. 1, Minneapolis, MN 55421).

Aerobicise: The Ultimate Workout—105 minutes of advanced workout for the person in shape.

American Health and Fitness of Body and Mind: Getting It All Back—Self-test aerobics, muscle strength, and flexibility.

The Beach Workout with David Essel—45 minutes of low-impact, high-energy aerobic conditioning.

Bodies in Motion II—includes two workouts: 30 minutes for beginners, 90 minutes for advanced exercisers.

Body by Diet Center—well-designed workouts with three intensity levels.

Body Focus—low-impact aerobics; beginner to intermediate.

Broadway Body—Warm-up, workout, cool-down.

Crystal Light National Aerobic Championship Workout—Warm-up, low-impact aerobic workout for beginners, and cool-down.

Dance Away—Warm-up, low-impact aerobics, cool-down.

Dance Away: Get Fit with the Hits—Warm-up, low-impact aerobics, cool-down, and stretch.

Fitness Formula with Judi Sheppard Missett—a safe and effective aerobic workout.

The Freedanse II Advantage with Suzy Stone—A balanced warm-up with a freedanse-style aerobic workout.

High Energy Aerobics: Joanie Greggins—warm-up, 12-minute continuous exercise, and cool-down.

Jane Fonda Challenge—90-minute workout; cardiac strength, tone, flexibility, and circulation.

Jane Fonda Prime Time Workout—50 minutes; cardiac strength, tone, flexibility, and circulation.

Jane's Complete Workout—
  Beginner
    low impact
    new exercises
    complete workout
    easy
  Intermediate
    low impact
    new exercises
    complete workout
    easy
    with weights
  Advanced
    workout challenge
    complete workout
    with weights

Jazzercise: Judi Sheppard Missett—aerobic workout; beginner to intermediate.

Kathy Smith's Starting Out—good workout for beginners.

Kathy Smith's Winning Workout—warm-up, aerobic workout with weights, cool-down; includes a 12-week weight-training program.

Martina—total body workout, fitness and training, warm-up stretch, cardiac agility, workout with weights, and post-workout stretch.

New York Aerobics—working out indoors and out.

No Jump Aerobics—warm-up with low impact aerobics, 20-minute workout, and cool-down.

No Stress Workout—includes high-energy workout and low-impact aerobics with light weights.

One on One with Linda Shelton—includes aerobics with and without weights and muscle-sculpting with progressive resistance.

Phil Simms Workout—workout with stretches, weight resistance, aerobics, and cool-down.

Rev Up with Charlene Prickett—high-energy workout.

Self-defense Aerobics—warm-up, aerobics with strength and energy workout, cool-down, and relaxation.

Stanford Health and Exercise Program—experts discuss training and health benefits with the use of cycling, tennis, golf, and swimming.

Start Up: Jane Fonda—25-minute exercise program with warm-up and low-impact aerobics.

20-Minute Workout—three workouts with aerobics, stretching, and fitness.

Glossary

Aerobic Literally means "with oxygen." Aerobic exercise utilizes oxygen in order to recycle ATP and in turn contract the working muscle.

Agonist muscle The muscle group that is the prime mover of contraction in an exercise.

Alignment The relationship of the body segments to one another.

Anaerobic Literally means "without oxygen." Anaerobic exercise recycles ATP and in turn contracts the working muscle without utilizing oxygen.

Anaerobic glycolysis The energy system that uses only the stored glycogen in our muscle cells to resynthesize ATP. This energy system is used for intense bursts of energy and can only last for the first 2 minutes of exercise.

Antagonist muscle The muscle group that opposes the prime mover (agonist) muscle. The antagonist muscle is usually stretched while the prime mover is contracted.

ATP (adenosine triphosphate) A substance that must be present in the muscle cell in order for the muscle to contract.

Ballistic stretch A stretch that utilizes body momentum to force the muscle groups into as much extensibility as can be tolerated.

Body composition The total of fat weight and lean body weight. The assessment of body composition determines the body's percentages of fat and lean weight.

Cardiac output The total amount of blood the heart pumps in one minute.

Cardiorespiratory endurance The ability of the cardiovascular system (heart and blood vessels) and the respiratory system (lungs and air passages) to function efficiently during sustained, vigorous activities (also called *cardiovascular endurance*).

Circuit training A specific exercise or routine that is performed in a given period of time. Once completed, a new exercise or routine is performed with a specific time frame. A series of these timed exercises is called a "circuit."

Creatine phosphate A phosphagen, similar to ATP, that is stored in the muscle cells and used as an immediate energy source for anaerobic activity.

Diastolic blood pressure A measure of the resting pressure in the arteries when the heart is not contracting.

Flexibility The range of motion of a certain joint and its corresponding muscle groups.

Glycogen   The storage form of glucose. It is found in large amounts in the muscle cells and the liver. It serves as an important source of energy during exercise.

Hemoglobin   A protein cell present in the blood that transports oxygen to the working muscle.

Interval training   Series of high-intensity exercises alternated with periods of rest.

Kilocalorie   The energy food releases measured in calories.

Kyphosis   A postural deviation where the muscles of the upper back are weakened and therefore develop a rounded or hunched appearance.

Lactic acid   The end product of anaerobic glycolysis. As lactic acid builds in a muscle cell, the muscle fatigues and muscular contraction becomes increasingly difficult.

Lordosis   An extreme forward tilt of the pelvic girdle. In this position, the abdominal muscles are overstretched and the lower back muscles are overcontracted (also called *swayback*).

Metabolism   The body's process of converting food into energy through numerous chemical reactions.

Muscular endurance   The ability of local skeletal muscles to perform work strenuously for progressively longer periods of time.

Overload principle   The ability of the body to adapt to higher performance levels and gradually increase its capacity to do more work.

Perceived exertion   A self-test used during the aerobic workout to detect signs of fatigue. The perceived exertion scale was formalized by Borg in 1982.

Phosphagen energy system   The energy system named after the presence of creatine phosphate, which exists in the muscle cells. The phosphagen energy system is utilized in the initial burst of energy for muscular contraction.

Placement   The relative positioning of the individual body parts.

Posture   The position of the body as it is held in space.

Progression   A gradual increase in the overload of a workout. Progression can be applied to the duration, intensity, or frequency of the workout.

Recovery heart rate   The heart rate 1 minute after exercise is stopped, which indicates how quickly you recover from exercise.

Resting heart rate   The heart rate taken just after waking up in the morning.

Somatotype   A system for classifying the three general body types: endomorph, mesomorph, and ectomorph.

Specificity principle   The ability of the body to adapt specifically to the demands placed on it.

Static stretch   A position of extreme stretch on a given muscle group that is assumed and held for a period of time.

Step workout   A type of aerobic conditioning that uses a low bench to perform specific exercises.

Strength   The ability of a muscle or group of muscles to exert a force against a resistance in one all-out effort.

Stroke volume   The amount of blood the heart pumps per beat.

Synergist muscle   The muscle group that assists but is not the prime mover (agonist) in an exercise.

Systolic blood pressure   A measure of the rhythmic contraction of the heart as blood leaves it through the ventricles. Systolic blood pressure rises with increased cardiac output.

Talk test   A method for measuring the intensity of an aerobic activity. You must be able to carry on a conversation during exercise or the intensity of the activity is too great.

Target heart rate   The rate at which your heart must work in order to affect your aerobic capacity (also called the *exercise heart rate*).

Tempo   The speed at which a piece of music is performed.

Threshold of training   The minimum amount of exercise necessary to produce improvements in physical fitness.

Training effect   The physiological changes that occur in the body due to regular and proper participation in a fitness program.

References

1. Allsen, Philip E. *Conditioning and Physical Fitness.* Dubuque, IA: Brown, 1978.
2. American College of Obstetricians and Gynecologists. *Exercise During Pregnancy and Postnatal Period.* Washington, DC: ACOG, 1985.
3. American College of Sports Medicine. "Recommendations and Quality of Exercise for Developing and Maintaining Fitness in Healthy Adults." *Journal of Physical Education and Recreation* 51, no. 5 (May 1980): 17–18.
4. Astrand, P., and K. Rodahl. *Textbook of Work Physiology.* New York: McGraw Hill, 1977.
5. Bailey, Covert. *Fit or Fat?* Boston: Houghton Mifflin, 1977.
6. Benson, Herbert. *The Relaxation Response.* New York: Avon, 1975.
7. Fahey, Thomas D. *Athletic Training: Principles and Practices.* Mountain View, CA: Mayfield, 1986.
8. Bogart, J., et al. *Nutrition and Physical Fitness.* Philadelphia: Saunders, 1979.
9. Bucher, Charles A., and William E. Prentice. *Fitness for College and Life.* St. Louis: Times/Mirror, Mosby, 1985.
10. Cantu, Robert C. *Sports Medicine in Primary Care.* Lexington, MA: Heath, 1982.
11. ———. *Clinical Sports Medicine.* Lexington, MA: Heath, 1983.
12. ———, and William Jay Gillespie. *Sports Medicine, Sports Science: Bridging the Gap.* Lexington, MA: Heath, 1982.
13. Clearly, Monica L., Robert J. Moffat, and Kathleen M. Knutzen. "The Effects of Two- and Three-Day per Week Aerobic Dance Programs on Maximal Oxygen Uptake." *Research Quarterly for Exercise and Sport* 55, no. 1(1984): 172–174.
14. Cooper, Kenneth H. *The Aerobics Way.* New York: Evans, 1977.
15. Corbin, Charles B., and Ruth Lindsey. *Concepts of Fitness.* Dubuque, IA: Brown, 1985.
16. ———. *Concepts of Physical Fitness with Laboratories.* Dubuque, IA: Brown, 1985.
17. Day, Nancy Raines. "Footowner's Manual: A Guide to Good Foot Care." *Shape Magazine* (July 1985).
18. DeVries, H. A. *Physiology of Exercise for Physical Education and Athletics,* 3d ed. Dubuque, IA: Brown, 1980.
19. Dintiman, George B., Stephen E. Stone, Jude C. Pennington, and Robert G. Davis. *Discovering Lifetime Fitness: Concepts of Exercise and Weight Control.* St. Paul, MN: West, 1984.

20. Dowdy, Deborah, Kirk J. Cureton, Harry P. DuVal, and Harvey G. Outz. "Effects of Aerobic Dance on Physical Work Capacity, Cardiovascular Function, and Body Composition of Middle-aged Women. *Research Quarterly for Exercise and Sport* 56, no. 3(1985): 227–233.

21. Dusek, Dorothy E. *Thin and Fat: Your Personal Lifestyle.* Belmont, CA: Wadsworth, 1978.

22. Falls, Harold B., Ann M. Baylor, and Rod K. Dishman. *Essentials of Fitness.* Philadelphia: SCP, 1980.

23. Fleck, Steven J., and William J. Kraemer. "The Overtraining Syndrome." *NSCA Journal* (August, September 1982).

24. Fox, Edward L., Richard W. Bowers, and Merle L. Foss. *The Physiological Basis of Physical Education and Athletics.* Philadelphia: Saunders, 1988.

25. Fox, S. M., J. P. Naughton, and W. L. Hackell. "Physical Activity: The Prevention of Coronary Heart Disease." *Annals of Clinical Research* 3 (1971): 404–432.

26. Francis, Kennon T. "Delayed Muscle Soreness: A Review." *Journal of Orthopedic and Sports Physical Therapy* (1983).

27. Francis, Lorna L. *Injury Prevention Manual for Dance Exercises.* San Diego, CA: National Injury Prevention Foundation, 1983.

28. Gelder, Naneene Van, ed. *Aerobic Dance— Exercise Instructor Manual.* San Diego: IDEA Foundation, 1987.

29. Getchell, Bud. *Physical Fitness: A Way of Life,* 3d ed. New York: Macmillan, 1983.

30. Goodman Kraines, Minda, and Esther Kan. *Jump into Jazz.* Palo Alto, CA: Mayfield, 1983.

31. Jacobson, Edmund. *You Must Relax.* New York: McGraw-Hill, 1962.

32. Jensen, Clayne R., and Garth A. Fisher. *Scientific Basis of Athletic Conditioning,* 2d ed. Philadelphia: Lea & Febiger, 1979.

33. Katch, F. I., and W. D. McArdle. *Nutrition, Weight Control, and Exercise.* Boston: Houghton Mifflin, 1977.

34. Kisselle, Judy, and Karen Mazzeo. *Aerobic Dance, Alternate Edition.* Englewood, CO: Morton, 1984.

35. Krepton, Dorie, and Donald Chu. *Everybody's Aerobic Book,* Edina, MN: Bellwether Press, 1986.

36. Lamb, David R. *Physiology of Exercise: Response and Adaptations,* 2d ed. New York: Macmillan, 1984.

37. Martin, B. J. "Effect of Warm-up on Metabolic Responses to Strenuous Exercise." *Medicine in Science and Sport* 7, no. 2(1975): 146–149.

38. McArdle, William D., Frank I. Katch, and Victor L. Katch. *Exercise Physiology: Energy, Nutrition, and Human Performance.* Philadelphia: Lea & Febiger, 1981.

39. Moorhouse, Laurence. *Total Fitness.* New York: Simon and Schuster, 1975.

40. Nash, Jay B. "You Must Relax—But How?" *Health Education* 16 (April–May 1985): 9–12.

41. Pollock, M. L., J. H. Wilmore, and S. M. Fox. *Exercise in Health and Disease.* Philadelphia: Saunders, 1984.

42. Rasch, P. J., and R. K. Burke. *Kinesiology and Applied Anatomy,* 6th ed. Philadelphia: Lea & Febiger, 1978.

43. Selye, Hans. *The Stress of Life.* New York: McGraw-Hill, 1956.

44. Sharkey, Brian J. *Physiology of Fitness.* Champaign, IL: Human Kinetics, 1979.

45. Simonson, Ernst, ed. *Physiology of Work Capacity and Fatigue.* Springfield, IL: Thomas, 1971.

46. University of California, Cardiac Rehabilitation Program. "Things to Know About Your Lower Back." Davis, CA: 1981.

47. Vitale, Frank. *Individualized Fitness Program.* Englewood Cliffs, NJ: Prentice-Hall, 1973.

48. White, J. R. "EKG Changes Using Carotid Artery for HR Monitoring." *Medicine and Science in Sports and Exercise* 9 (1977): 88–94.

49. Williams, Melvin. *Lifetime Physical Fitness.* Dubuque, IA: Brown, 1985.

Index